AMBER WOULD LIKE ᴛᴏ ...

There are many important people in my life that I am so happy to know and have supporting me on this journey.

First and foremost, thank you to my parents, Brian and Linda, for believing in me and my vision for my business and career. Thank you for always giving me the freedom to create and live a passionate life, and the courage to begin on the path to achieving my biggest goals and dreams.

To my father, this would not be possible without your support and inspiration. You have my admiration for having the best work ethic of anyone I've ever known. I'm so glad I inherited that from you. The support you've given me as a father has been, without a doubt, the most priceless and loving actions a father could give to his daughter. I will forever hold this deeply in my heart.

To Teresa de Grosbois for your coaching and support with helping me to get this book off the ground, for believing in me enough to play a big game of influence in my business, as well as for being such a powerful woman of knowledge. You truly inspire me.

To Frank Moffatt for lighting the fire under my ass to set a date to get the writing done for this book to be a reality for me much sooner than I had anticipated becoming an Author. Also thank you for your coaching and support on this journey.

Thank you to Lisa D. Martinez for doing such a fabulous job of editing the content for this book, correcting my spelling errors, and making it sound even more delicious than it already is! You are such a talented woman!

To Jeff Fraser for helping me to design the book while having a ridiculously busy work schedule. I am so excited that you helped me to bring my vision to life. I know this is setting the stage for the birth, and growth, of the massive wave of Amber Approved branding to come!

To Perry Thompson, such a gifted and talented photographer, for taking the beautiful photos for the recipes. Your generosity and support is so deeply appreciated and I am so honored to have you as a part of this, and many more books to come.

Thanks to all my taste-testers for giving honest feedback and suggestions after creating over 60 recipes over the last few months! Tanya, Jill, Alaina, Jackie, Becky, Lisa, Theresa, Jaclyn, Kassandra, Shannon, Kaley and Tessa—thanks so much for Approving of my Amber Approved creations.

And a very dear thank you for everyone else, including all my friends and family, for your involvement and for believing in me and my vision for this book as well as your continued love and support. It is with all my heart that I thank you and I am so humbled to have you all in my life.

FOREWARD

Rice and plain chicken. It's June 2001 and I have lost over 50 pounds for inability to keep food down. Rice and plain chicken are the only two foods I know I can eat. The Doctors have done test after test and now they are simply telling me I can't digest certain foods.

Big surprise. I've known that for months. As a recovering food addict, I am not sure whether to be happy or devastated at the news.

Far from being doomed to a life of dull and boring foods, I have now discovered that gluten-free, corn free, dairy-free, sugar-free cooking not only tastes better but has me far more energized and active. Bonus - when I eat right my emotions don't run rampant and I need a lot less sleep.

Enter my hero. Amber Romaniuk, who I can honestly say has put some of the yummiest, healthiest food I have ever tasted in front of me.

"Amber Approved" was created by Amber, owner of Nourish This Life. Like me, she went through a vicious cycle of emotional eating and food addiction, and, subsequently, discovered how certain foods have a massive negative impact on her body physically, mentally, and emotionally. The biggest culprits were refined sugar and any products containing gluten or dairy. Who knew?

This book, will be the first of many editions to come. (Those of us who love Amber's cooking just aren't willing to live with only one of these). Amber is brilliant at combining ingredients so you can enjoy healthy varieties of your favourite recipes without compromising flavour, appeal, or quality. These recipes use top-quality whole-food ingredients that satisfy without creating powerful, distracting cravings. There's even some whole new recipe ideas that you will love.

This book was made so Amber can show you it is possible to make healthy changes without feeling like you are on a "diet" or having to cut out your favourite foods. You will learn how to live a life of freedom and balance away from the eating issues that once seemed unstoppable.

You'll get some of Amber's favourites, with over 60 recipes including my favourites, pumpkin spice cookies, chocolate avocado pudding, egg salad rolls, paleo turkey burgers and banana bread French toast, all of which, by the end of this sentence, have made my mouth begin to water. There is also a wide range of suggestions for using healthy alternatives for the recipes in this book so you won't feel like you don't have enough options to create. The possibilities are endless when it comes to experimenting with healthy options.

These recipes will benefit those who want to avoid gluten, sugar, dairy, MSG, aspartame, corn, and soy. The recipes are also supportive of better blood sugar balance, easier on digestion, and free of the most common food allergens, which are dairy and wheat. They will also open up your mind to using ingredients in a way that you may not have thought possible—like using avocados to make a creamy and satisfying chocolate pudding. Wow! Just try it. You'll love it.

Teresa de Grosbois
Chair, Evolutionary Business Council

Teresa de Grosbois is a word of mouth marketing expert, 3X best selling author, international speaker and founder of the Evolutionary Business Council.

AMBER

(APPROVED

GLUTEN, SUGAR & DAIRY-FREE RECIPES TO NOURISH THIS LIFE

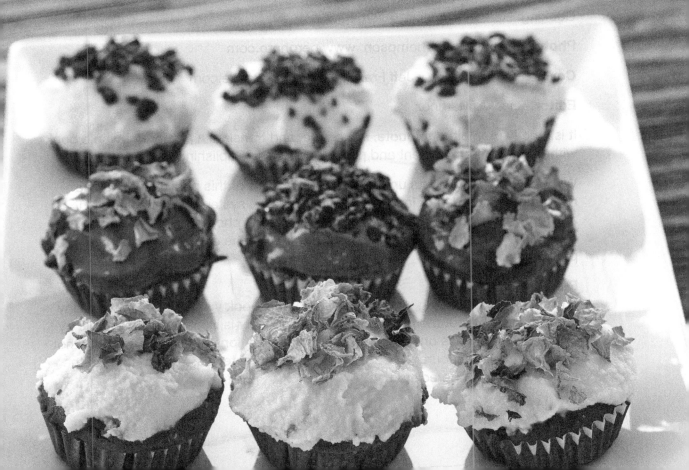

NOURISH THIS LIFE

Amber Approved
Gluten, Sugar & Dairy-Free Recipes to Nourish This Life
Written by Amber Romaniuk

Copyright © 2013
By Amber Romaniuk

Published by Nourish This Life
Calgary, Canada

www.nourishthislife.ca | amber@nourishthislife.ca

All Rights Reserved

ISBN: 978-0-9936238-0-6

Health, Fitness: Nutrition
Cooking / Healthy & Healing / Gluten-Free
Cooking: Health & Healing- Allergy

Photographs - Perry Thompson, www.perphoto.com

Cover & Book Design - Jeff Fraser, www.otherorange.com

Editor - Lisa D. Martinez

CONTENTS

RECIPES

Breakfast

Dips & Dressings

Side Dishes & Salads, Soups & The Main Event

Sweets, Treats & Desserts

INTRODUCTION

In a day and age where there are so many questions about food and nutrition—what to eat and what to stay away from—it can seem very intimidating if you are new to making lifestyle changes when it comes to food.

Two common questions are:

Where do I start? What are the more natural options?

The answers? By investing in this book, you have already begun, and there are so many options available these days that with the direction provided within these pages, you will be headed down the right path.

I also hear complaints such as:

Won't it taste like cardboard?

It doesn't have to. That is a common misconception. Good food doesn't have to taste bad. It sometimes takes trial and error to get it right, but that's where I come in—I have done that for you, taking the guess work out of healthy, delicious food. Just because you are shifting to a healthier, nutrient-dense way of eating, doesn't mean you have to sacrifice your favourite foods.

That is why I'm so excited to share this first book with you—to show you it's not only possible to enjoy delicious ingredients without feeling deprived, without sacrificing taste, and without feeling guilty for indulging a little, but it can be easy too. I want to inspire you to experiment and enjoy cooking and baking while trying new ingredients without fear and apprehension. I hope to help you create a whole new relationship with your food and yourself.

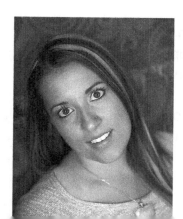

MY STORY

Why gluten, sugar, and dairy-free?

It's a story that has been long in the making, starting at about the age of five for me.

It was the first day of attending school from a new house on a beautiful acreage my parents had just built. The air was crisp, and the leaves had begun to turn colour as fall was on its way. There were all sorts of emotions and anticipation running through my gut as I waited for the bus to arrive. I felt butterflies, excitement, and nervousness. Would the kids be nice? Who would I sit with? I was excited to make new friends on the bus ride to school.

As it stopped in front of me, my heart started to beat rapidly against my chest. There were so many older kids, but it was the older boys—mean boys—that stood out the most. They began to taunt me. Laughter rang out like shots to my very soul. They called me fat. Ugly.

I was five years old.

Although I didn't realize it then, my world was being created in that image. The image of a fat, ugly little girl that didn't belong. I was crushed. I felt ruined. I was shocked that anyone would be so mean to someone they didn't even know. All of the excitement and light inside of me was replaced with sadness and a feeling that I wasn't good enough—all before I could even sit down. I didn't want to be on that bus. I wanted to be with my mom or my dad instead. They would never hurt me like that.

This experience created, and then shaped, many of the patterns and actions that I would carry through for the next twenty years of my life. From a young age I became very self-conscious about my body and felt as though I was unlovable by the opposite sex. Hearing I was fat hurt me deeply.

I was raised by amazing parents, and they gave me so much love, but with strangers and people I wasn't familiar with, I was very shy and tended to take time to come out of my shell. It all started with that one experience on the bus.

I grew up consuming the typical Standard American Diet. To give some insight, perhaps you recall a nutritional guideline of sorts, or those silly food pyramids given at school when we were young that preached which foods we were to eat, and how many servings a day. Eating tons of breads, cereals, and pastas was emphasized, as well as plenty of dairy, fruits, vegetables, and meat for protein.

Well, I definitely ate tons of wheat and dairy, a bit of meat, and a few fruits and vegetables, but my favourite food group was sugar. Ice cream, doughnuts, sugary cereals, chocolate bars, candy—you name it, if it had sugar, it was my favourite. I didn't care much for vegetables, at least not unless they were swimming in cheese or butter.

Growing up, my mother and I shared a close relationship. She was very loving and nurturing and a big part of the relationship we shared together was food. We'd go out to eat or go to the store where I could pick whatever I wanted—cookies, cakes, candy, chocolate bars—I was always consuming something with sugar, but it was like a reward, it was always fun to share with my mother. My father and I also shared a close relationship, but it was based more on activities like learning to ski, quad, and sea-doo.

I was always a bit more on the pudgy side growing up, and again, I got the odd comment here or there from guys at school. I, of course, took this personally and it further verified what the boys on the bus had said that first day. It must have been true since it was still happening, all the way through junior high and high school. I thought since my mother was overweight (and her side of the family was overweight) that I'd inherited her genes. I believed that I too would always be a bit on the bigger side. It made sense.

I was not aware that the things I was putting into my body would make that big of an impact. I had no confidence. I was shy. I was too scared to talk to boys for fear of being hurt. I created the story that I wasn't good enough, I was not lovable, I was chubby and ugly, and that was that.

Humans are social creatures and we will find a relationship where we can, if not from someone, then from something. Substances, reckless activities, alcohol—for me it was food. So, the relationship I had with food grew. It was always there. It never disappointed. It always made me happy. Being surrounded by an endless amount of delicious, beautiful, sweet-looking foods brought me so much joy. I was always excited, so much that almost every memory I had created in my life had some association with food. It was like I could eat AND go swimming, eat AND celebrate Christmas, eat AND watch television.

There were always plenty of goodies to gorge on. The light came back brighter when I could enjoy my favourite foods and an activity. Another one of the habits I created was eating while watching television and movies. Eating junk food, sweets, or fast food while being distracted by the television was a habit that my parents and I shared together. We bonded while being distracted together, and eating. This was what love looked like to me. Little did I realize, down the road, this would be a large obstacle for me to overcome.

Once I hit high school, I wanted more attention and I started to change. I was learning how to come into my beauty and I started yo-yo dieting. I decided to try to eat better, a few extra vegetables, less cheese and sugar. I ate smaller portions and lost ten pounds really quickly, only to go back to my old habits. It became a rollercoaster. I never liked my weight, it was always too high of a number, and I developed a lack of self-worth because of it. I saw other girls in school that were skinnier and got more attention. They had boyfriends and it made me jealous. I was so far away from self-love and acceptance, but was getting more caught up in having a better body image because I thought that was the only way I'd get guys to like me. I didn't even know what self-love or acceptance meant.

After graduating high school I moved to Calgary, Canada to attend the Southern Alberta Institute of Technology (SAIT) for Broadcast News. I wanted to be on television. Once college started I felt like I had a new start. New city, new people, new everything and I felt like I could create more of a state of acceptance. My classmates and I quickly bonded, although, my nutrition definitely didn't get better upon leaving my parents' house and living in Calgary. I'd try to buy a few vegetables, but it was still full of garbage foods, and now since I was legal, lots of drinking. Partying was a huge part of the college lifestyle, followed by eating poorly all the time because it was convenient and our school schedule was so busy. There were plenty of trips to fast food restaurants and our building's little café for dinners of ice cap latte's and chocolate puffed wheat squares.

In December of 2005 I started to get random stomach pains, cramps and bloating, but I ignored it for a while, thinking it was nothing. But when it started to get bad, especially after eating really poorly, I went to the doctor. She diagnosed me with Irritable Bowel Syndrome, told me to eat less bread and that I would be fine. Time passed and I didn't change much, even though I felt pain more often. I loved my sweets, junk food, and drinking far too much to ever give them up.

Eventually, I got a second opinion from a Holistic Doctor. She shared that I had Candida, an overgrowth of bad bacteria in my gut, and this was creating my symptoms of bloating, pain, and constant cravings for sugar and refined foods. She advised the Candida diet for a few weeks, consisting of eating nothing but vegetables, eggs, meat, fish, and brown rice. I didn't care much, attempted the diet for two days and gave up. It was far too strict and I missed my comfort foods. This would be one of many future attempts of this diet for me to come.

Stress from a relationship created other health issues, and it was when my ex-boyfriend broke up with me that I started to calm down, relieve the stress and come back to myself. Before this happened I was hoping the doctors in the Western medical system could help me, but none of them could. They all wanted to put me on 1 of 25 prescription drugs and could not explain my symptoms. It was gifted Natural Health practitioners that were able to get me to the root of my health concerns.

Once I got my heart broken, I was determined to get him back, so I made the commitment to change my habits and lose weight. If I was skinnier and more beautiful, how could he resist me, right? Initially, because of the hurt I felt, I wasn't hungry. All the love that had filled my heart, and me, was disappearing because the relationship was broken, and instead, a void appeared. I had to force myself to eat, and it was tiny amounts. I lost 7 pounds in 2 weeks and was motivated to keep going. I started to exercise and felt great relief from it. I had a spark in me from the heartache that I felt such a high after exercise, and I started to notice a difference. So did everyone else. My appetite didn't grow, but my exercise routine did, and I lost another 7 pounds in 2 weeks. I was ecstatic.

My goal was to get to 125 pounds and I felt like if I did this, I'd have conquered the world and would get my boyfriend back. The closer I got to my goal, the more I deprived myself to get there, eating only a set number of calories a day. Extreme guilt filled my mind and body if I ate too much, or consumed foods I wasn't allowed. I would become disappointed in myself for not being perfect. I would scold myself on the inside, "Amber, how could you, shame on you, you're so stupid for doing that."

It was like I was committing a crime and no one was to know I did this, as I was striving for perfection, and didn't want anyone to think of me as less than that. I was working out 2 hours a day, 6 days a week and thought I looked and felt great, but it was hard to maintain. The drill sergeant in my head would scold me and yell at me to work harder when I had overindulged. "Do you want to be fat again? You won't reach your goals eating like a pig." That voice was such an ass all the time.

As summer came, I went to a barbecue and had decided before I got there that I wasn't eating any of the ice cream cake I was bringing, or any food other than a salad. I didn't want to gain a pound, only keep losing to reach 125. Instead of watching what I ate, I gorged on everything from burgers to cake, and ate WAY too much. Then, I decided I would barely eat the next day and workout harder to compensate. Soon after, the pattern of bingeing and then depriving to compensate was created. I met my goal of 125 pounds. The bad news, my boyfriend didn't want me back. I felt as if I'd failed, and even though I looked perfect physically, I still wasn't good enough. I was crushed again and felt like I was that little girl on the bus all over again. My efforts felt like they were for nothing. I was so lonely and my void was getting bigger. My attitude became that if he wasn't going to love me with this hot new bod, then screw it, it wasn't worth it. I'd rather eat.

This is where my vicious cycle of bingeing really grabbed hold. I would just allow myself to cheat on everything I was craving. It turned into full days of me driving around the city buying all these foods I desired that would make me happy. I deserved it, I needed the love and the comfort since I was broken-hearted. I made the rounds to everything from Subway, to specialty cupcake stores, chocolates, or heading to the grocery store to buy 2 or 3 bags of junk food. Then I would go home and binge while watching television. I was completely distracted and numb from my reality, my emotions, and lack of self-love. I would probably consume anywhere between 4000 to 8000 calories on a binge day or evening, but I didn't care.

The more I did this, the worse the cravings and my appetite got, I became unhappier. Because now I was in pain, mentally and physically, and gaining weight like crazy. I gained 50 pounds in 4 months. I was ashamed and I isolated myself because I didn't want people to see how I used to look so thin and was now so fat, that was complete self-defeat and sabotage in my eyes.

I was so angry. I blamed my ex, I blamed everything and everyone for what I was doing to myself. I would eat so much, be so bloated, and in so much pain that it was awful. But the cravings, and my mentality, overpowered me. I just kept doing it. I'd binge for a few days, then deprive myself, then get really hungry, get a craving and binge.

It was my secret world that no one knew about, and no one was ever to know about. I would eat so much and throw the rest in the garbage, but then a couple of hours later, I would go digging for it and eat more when I had room. It was my living hell. I was so ashamed, and addicted. I had hit my low. I never envisioned myself digging through my garbage to eat more. Disgusting. I felt worthless, I hated myself, I was humiliated, and I had no idea how I would be able to stop myself. I didn't allow myself to have fun or go out and enjoy time with my friends because I was too fat and unworthy of enjoyment anymore.

After a year I realized I was being extremely unhealthy and wanted to change my ways. I started to clean up my diet slowly. I'd have one cheat day a week, and got back into exercising. The weight slowly started to come off. On my cheat day, I would still binge hard, and I still felt guilty afterward. It was difficult to get rid of my cravings after my cheat day. But this was my all-out day to gorge on my favourite foods.

After about 6 months I dropped from 175 to 145 pounds and it felt great. I was still obsessed with a lower number and wanted to be 125 to 130 pounds again. I was never satisfied with my weight. I would lose a few more pounds, hit 135, but then a trigger would hit, like having a bad day, or eating one bad thing, and that would be it.

It was like a switch in my brain would flip on and there was no stopping me. I would spend so much time fantasizing and obsessing about the foods that I would buy after work that nothing else occupied my mind. I had a bad day and I deserved some comfort. I would spend so much money on the food, go home and begin my pig fest. Those first few bites were like pure ecstasy. I felt so happy, like I was on a high. I felt relief, comfort, and a calmness come over me as I ate that brownie, muffin, ice cream, and cookies. I looked around me and saw the surrounding mass of food, popped in my movie, and felt like I could escape away. Nothing mattered, and I felt nothing, for that time because I was numb from my emotions.

The vicious cycle hadn't really stopped, but it was less often. I began to cut out more, as I began to read and research about food quality, nutrition, and how certain foods could be almost addictive-like. First were dairy and alcohol, as I wasn't really a fan of dairy anymore and didn't want the empty calories from drinking. I'd make more poor food choices if I was drinking, and this would completely derail me, and for now, I didn't want that. I also read more about Candida and the foods that fed it, and alcohol was one of the worst culprits. Others included sugar, refined carbohydrates, yeast, and even dairy.

I also tried every diet. No dairy, Vegan, Vegetarian, just drinking smoothies, just eating salads, fasting, low carb. You name it, I've pretty much tried it all.

SPRING 2012

Attempting to cut out sugar and gluten was an extremely difficult struggle. I'd be successful for a few days, then crave them and binge. After more reading, there was evidence that suggested gluten and sugar had addictive qualities like heroin and meth. Not only was I psychologically in pain, but I had a food addiction, which added to the vicious cycle. The more I consumed, the more I would have to consume next time to get the same blissful high, before crashing and burning. After reading more about sugar and gluten addiction I felt relief that I wasn't crazy and I was addicted to these foods. I knew I could overcome this addiction, but it would take dedication and hard work to do so. If I could cut the addictive foods, my binges would be over, and I'd be free. I'd go back and forth and gain and lose the same 15 pounds over and over, this wasn't good for my mind, body, or anything.

I was fed up with the awful cravings and committed to fully give up processed sugars and gluten—for my health, and for my sanity. I figured if I felt the need to binge I'd rather eat too much fruit, nuts or smoothies than have to deal with the awful temptations of gluten and sugar.

At first it was extremely difficult, but I kept going. After a few months, my cravings for gluten, sugar, and refined carbs started to go away and I wasn't binging as often because of it. My moods were getting better. I noticed that consuming gluten and sugar made me in an almost depressed-like state, feeling worthless, guilty, and in pain. It would always take at least 5 or 6 days for these feelings to subside and for me to feel more like myself again.

SUMMER 2012

I had realized I needed to let go of the pattern of bingeing, and this would be my biggest challenge yet. I was told by someone that if I could let go of this, I would really be able to open up and become extremely in tune with my body, which would, in the future, help me with my career.

I really wanted this for myself and I had to try. After cutting out sugar and gluten I realized that my problem was actually on a psychological level, with the bingeing and emotional eating, because I still wanted to binge on healthy foods. I was still trying to fill a void, and bingeing was familiar, comfortable and no one could take that away from me. I could hide in shame and eat away all my fears, worries, doubts, insecurities, sadness, and anger in the forms of a dozen muffins, pancakes, smoothies, a bag of nuts—whatever I craved—a bag of brown rice pasta and a container of goat cheese, I'd stuff myself so full until I felt sick.

I wanted to stop, but the feelings were far too strong, and now I had created intense food sensitivities to these healthy foods I was bingeing on, which made me want to consume them even more. In the end I created more havoc. After doing more reading, I discovered when you create food sensitivity, on many levels, your body makes you crave this food even more. This completely made sense, but I had a whole new crop of foods to cut out, since I had been binging on them excessively and was now addicted and sensitive to them.

I was up and down from 135 to 150 again within a few weeks. I knew I had to stop. I knew my body was extremely sensitive and unhappy with me, and I was scared that continuing this behaviour of self-hate would eventually kill me. I didn't want that, I had too much amazing life to create for myself.

One evening, I went online and started doing research on eating disorders. I found websites, blogs, and videos of tons of people, mostly women, who were dealing with the same thing as me or had overcome their disorder. Seeing how common this was made me feel better, like I was not alone. I was also saddened to see how many others were struggling with the same hell I was.

Reading some of the blogs of women who were in their recovery from binge, emotional, compulsive eating, anorexia, and bulimia inspired me. If they could do it, there wasn't any reason I couldn't. I had to really help myself. A big part of that stepping stone forward was to share with others what I was dealing with and get some support, this was not something I wanted to do on my own.

I saw a psychologist once and that helped somewhat. Then, I found seeing a Medical Intuitive helped me so much because she was able to interpret what my body was trying to tell me, but I couldn't understand yet. I told my best friend and a few others, and I felt a bit better. I wanted to love myself, and when I realized that bingeing was self-hate, I really didn't want to do it anymore. If I wanted to truly love myself, I would have to stop this destructive behaviour that was running my life.

After going through a cleanse, and ending some shaky relationships, I needed comfort and chose to turn to food. The whole time I thought I was "in control" I wasn't. I was so afraid to lose control that I was living in fear the whole time thinking, "I wonder which day will be the day I let go and tumble back down."

Your thoughts create your future, so I believe, and my thoughts of losing control became my reality. This time I was devastated, as I had been sure I'd released the demon for good. But it was still about body image, compulsion, and escaping myself, which was easier than facing emotions and reality.

This time around, I accepted that I had more to learn before I could be rid of bingeing for good. So I allowed myself to sit in it and observe because I wanted to learn why I was doing this, so I could know how to let go of it for good. Food was not my enemy, and I was creating it to be a bad thing when it's a means of survival. It should be enjoyed, to a healthy extent.

Being in the clear, and then falling back in really made me realize how using food as a coping mechanism didn't serve me any longer. I finally had the courage to share my story with the people I truly cared about, and with the world, because this time, for real, I was ready to take responsibility for my life, my health, well-being, and sanity—to choose to love myself.

I was sick and tired of making myself sick and tired, bloated, in pain, and falling so far off track from who I really was, that it would take weeks or months to get back to me. My body deserved better.

I had realized it came down to me choosing: ignoring overwhelm, ignoring feelings, getting too busy and deciding, "I need a break, an escape, a disconnect from myself and I want to stop feeling all these feelings and numb myself."

I'd learned that I'd wanted to escape myself a lot, and did it so much that I would gain and lose my connection with myself over and over, which I was learning was the most valuable relationship in my life. The self-love and care disappeared when I chose food and, to me, was like hurting an innocent puppy. I would never do that, so why would I choose to continually hurt myself? I chose fear over love, and I had been suffering alone inside.

Along with directly dealing with reality and my emotions, I started to eat in a different way. Although, at first, I didn't have much of a choice. All my stomach could handle were steamed vegetables, meat, eggs, and some healthy fat like avocado and coconut milk. I had put my digestive system through so much hell that it was like a war zone and had had enough.

Accepting this was hard, but I was determined. I wanted to re-balance my poor gut as it had become so sensitive and, as per my vow to love myself, I wanted to heal mentally and physically. The thought of cutting out everything that would agitate my digestion upset me—no fruit, no nuts, no gluten-free muffins, no brown rice—it made me sad. But it wasn't really making ME sad, it was making the little crazy person in my head sad, because I would no longer be giving in, going through the highs and the lows. I'd be heading toward a state of balance. That little voice in my head would throw a fit like a little five-year-old kid, but I wouldn't give in, not anymore.

I read a really cool article on how to help re-balance the digestive system and it mentioned eating 3 well-balanced meals with good portions of proteins, carbs, and fat. This would help my intestinal lining to repair, reduce my cravings, and keep me satiated between meals. The thought of eating steamed vegetables all day was not appealing, but I had to try. It wouldn't be forever. The first week sucked, plain and simple. I craved nuts and fruit so bad, and had a headache, but refused to give up. It got a bit easier the next week, and so on, and the best part was, I wasn't binging! I had no desire anymore whatsoever. The combination of directly dealing with emotions and staying satisfied with my meals was making a huge difference in my life.

FALL 2012

I started to feel freedom, like it was working. Through cutting out the things I craved, my body was able to open up and crave things it really wanted like a fresh salad, home-made guacamole, or a thick, juicy bison steak! I became aware of my triggers, or what I liked to call my "red flags" and I stayed away from them the best that I could.

Starting the R.H.N. Holistic Nutrition program at the Canadian School of Natural Nutrition in the fall of 2012 also helped, as it fed my passions, I was learning more and I was busier, in a healthy way, feeding my body, mind, and soul with knowledge instead of food.

This made me happy, and in my heart I could feel how good I was going to be at school and with my career. I realized why I was put through this hell. All of this happened so I could come out on the other side with a purpose, a gift. A gift to understand the vicious cycles that psychological voids, food addictions, and emotional eating patterns can create—such destructive behaviour, but it can be overcome with a great support system, addressing the root cause and re-balancing the body, mind, and soul. I understand what others are going through with their issues around food because I went through it myself. I was a victim to addicting foods, body image, and then creating destructive behaviours that took over my life.

Now I have been able to add in a lot of amazing whole foods that I have come to love. Can you believe I had never tried a fresh pear until this year? This is because the only memory I had of them before was trying the canned variety in sugary syrup as a child, and hating them. Organic, fresh pears are amazing, like candy, nature's candy. I eat a variety of fruits, tons of vegetables, proteins like bison, chicken and turkey, eggs, tons of avocado, coconut and flax milk, flax and hemp seed, and a variety of other clean foods that keep me completely satiated and without negative cravings. I guess it's similar in some ways to Paleo, but I do still add in gluten-free grains like quinoa, brown rice, teff, and amaranth, which I love also.

Every day I am able to add something back in, because the psychological

cravings are gone. I don't feel like I don't have enough anymore because I have plenty of everything. Plenty of love, food, happiness. My stomach and digestive system also feel better every day thanks to my self-love and dedication.
This has also allowed me to add foods back in that I haven't had in ages like bananas, gluten-free muffins, raw chocolate and goat cheese, which I no longer crave and can eat on a regular basis and maintain my control.

It's no one's fault, and I blame no one. It's just taken time for me to go through it all, learn, and realize for myself why it was happening—to become aware it's not love. And I wanted to love me. I didn't want to disconnect from myself or be numb anymore. I wanted to be present in every part of my life. FEEL feelings and emotions…and the rain on my skin, the warmth of the sun. I wanted to feel love with myself, a connection I've been longing for my whole life that now I can give to me.

That's what I wanted and that's what I'm giving myself now.

I want a lot for my life: a successful career, endless self-growth and learning, many adventurous memories, a loving relationship with a man, kids one day, to be genuinely happy, and to be free from food and body-image being the focus of my world. I want to treat myself with love, care, and create a nurturing environment where I can fill my void with passion, love, and things I love.

Now I continue to move forward. Listening to my body and treating my intuition as my own best friend. My intuition has grown, and is another gift that is serving me more and more each day. Now I listen to the best friend in me, rather than the voice in my head that would sabotage me over and over. I want to continue to learn and grow, to keep on this healthy path and open my life to all of the opportunity that is headed my way.

There is so much I can offer this world and I can't wait to keep moving forward and enjoying life. I can't wait to sit down with my clients and create a space where they can be open, honest, and feel comfortable, where there is nothing to hide.

This is my journey and I am finally creating the courage to be open and share this. Living the beautiful, fulfilling life that I was born to live lights me up inside now.

I create a foundation of confidence, passion, love, power, knowledge, and nourishment. I am not scared or ashamed to tell my story anymore. It has opened the door to create a safe space for others to share their story, which is another gift to me, as it has made me realize how many people close to me have gone through, or are going through, similar things, and that I have inspired them to want to improve their own quality of life. Being told I'm an inspiration feels really amazing.

I wanted the opportunity to show you that no matter what you are dealing with, or what you have gone through, you can always create courage and choose to take a different path this time—one full of love and power instead of fear.

So now that I've found my balance, even through making this book, I have really seen how my relationship with myself and what I eat has shifted so much over the past few years. I never would I have dreamed that I would be able to be free of deprivation and creating all of these beautiful, delicious recipes to share with the world.

My experience has deeply inspired me to show others you can live a life of love and freedom from deprivation and guilt, and enjoy your favourite foods without sacrificing for poor nutrition and the feelings of guilt and shame.

INGREDIENTS TO ENJOY

Eggs
Fruits
Gluten-Free Flours & Grains
Healthy Fats

Meats
Natural Sweeteners
Nuts, Seeds & Nut Butters
Vegetables

INGREDIENTS TO AVOID

Aspartame
Corn
Dairy
Gluten
MSG

Refined Sugars
Processed Foods
Soy
Dairy

By all means, if you only want to go gluten-free and aren't ready to cut out dairy or sugar, take things one step at a time. Some people are able to go cold-turkey and replace things quickly, while others need one thing at a time to avoid becoming overwhelmed and then giving up.

Often we do not realize we are sensitive to something until we have eliminated it from our diet. It is common that once you have made the shift to using more natural ingredients, if you fall back and have something more refined, you will almost immediately notice the negative impact it has on your body physically, mentally, and emotionally.

Enjoy local fruits and vegetables; fresh nuts and seeds; free-range, grass-fed, and organic meat and eggs; and gluten-free grains. Moderate the amounts of sweet treats you indulge in. Although the recipes for indulgence offered within these pages are much healthier, moderation is still important. Once you are in tune with your body it's much easier to identify what may be causing imbalances like blood sugar spikes, energy lulls, and digestive issues. The body is very good at telling us what it needs, and when we take the time to tune in and listen, we can give it exactly what it desires. It's a practice that takes time to build, but it's 100% possible to do!

AMBER APPROVED INGREDIENTS

So, now that you are ready to try experimenting with new ingredients, let me share some of the amazing nutritional content of a few of the ingredients used in many of the recipes. Some of them you may not have heard of, but that's okay. We are on this journey of learning and discovery together, and this is your opportunity to try new things!

DAIRY-FREE ALTERNATIVES

Almond Milk

Brown Rice Milk

Coconut Milk

Coconut Almond Milk

Flax Milk

Hemp Milk

Oat Milk

Almond Yogurt

Coconut Yogurt

Coconut Ice Cream

Plant-based Protein Powders

GLUTEN-FREE GRAINS

Amaranth

Brown Rice

Brown Rice pasta

Buckwheat

Certified Gluten-Free Oats & Steel Cut Oats *(be sure to check the brand and make sure they aren't cross-contaminated with any glutinous crops)*

Millet

Quinoa & Quinoa Flakes

Quinoa Pasta

Quinoa & Brown Rice Pasta

Teff

GLUTEN-FREE FLOURS

All Purpose Blend

Almond Flour

Amaranth Flour

Arrowroot Flour

Brown Rice Flour

Certified Gluten-Free Oat Flour

Chickpea Flour

Coconut Flour

Potato Flour

Quinoa Flour

Tapioca Flour

Teff Flour

AMBER APPROVED INGREDIENTS

HEALTHY FATS

Avocados & Avocado Oil

Camalina Oil

Coconut Butter

Unrefined Virgin Coconut Oil

Grapeseed Oil

Olive Oil

Raw Nuts & Nut Butters:
Almonds, Cashews, Hazelnuts, Macadamia Nuts, Pecans and Walnuts

Seeds: Chia, flax, hemp, sunflower and pumpkin seeds

NATURAL SWEETENERS

Apple Sauce

*Artichoke Syrup

Bananas

Blackstrap Molasses

Coconut Palm Sugar

Coconut Palm Nectar

*Lucuma Powder

Medjool Dates or Date Paste

Pure Dark-Grade Maple Syrup

Raw Unpasteurized Honey

Stevia

*Yacon Syrup

FRUITS & VEGETABLES

The more colour on your plate, the more nutrients you are getting. Seeing green, purple, yellow, orange, and red not only appeals to the eye, but also the health. Each colour represents different vitamins and minerals that your body needs to stay in balance.

Supporting local Farmers' Markets, as well as organic markets, as much as possible is the way to go. When you buy from your local Farmers, you are able to ask questions like where your food is coming from, if they spray with pesticides, or what they add to the soil. If it's not possible for you to buy all organic, all the time, consider switching the most pesticide-laden fruits and vegetables which include apples, bell peppers, strawberries, grapes, cucumbers, celery, spinach and bell peppers to organic options. Then, if necessary, the rest you can get elsewhere.

*NOTE

Here is a bit of information on some of the ingredients that may be less well-known and what they are good for in recipes.

*Artichoke Syrup is a low-glycemic sweetener that has a cross flavor between maple syrup and blackstrap molasses. It contains pre-biotics, which help to feed the healthy bacteria in our large intestine. It's also great for gut health!

*Lucuma Powder is a low-glycemic sweetener that comes from the lucuma fruit that has been dried and ground into a powder. It has a bit of a maple or caramel taste and is great for any icing, ice-cream, pudding or sweet-style recipe.

*Yacon Syrup is a low-glycemic dark syrup that is great in place of maple syrup or honey for any baking, icings, puddings or ice-creams.

*Maca Powder is a plant root originating from Peru. It is said to help support energy levels, stamina, fertility and enhanced libido. It has a bit of a bitter chocolate flavor and blends well with any chocolate recipe.

BASIC TIPS FOR COOKING & BAKING

1. Don't be afraid to experiment and make different versions of the same recipe. Add in extra spices or ingredients if you want. For example, instead of just chocolate avocado pudding you could add organic peppermint extract for a peppermint version. Once you have the basics down, it's really easy to make many different versions of a recipe.

2. Don't get stressed out about following the recipe 100%. When we put stress into a recipe, we are adding an energy that may make it not turn out as well. If we are more carefree and having fun in the kitchen instead, it usually turns out better than we could ever expect! (Like when your mom said her special ingredient was love, it was as if you could taste the love that went into the recipe.)

3. Get your family involved and make it a ritual once a week that everyone gets together to help in the kitchen and learn something they didn't know before. It can be as simple as using Lucuma powder for the first time, or making their first batch of Banana Bread French Toast!

4. Have some key ingredients available all the time. It's always a good idea to have a nice selection of fruits, veggies, nuts and seeds, eggs, flours, sweeteners, dairy-free milks, spices, and meats on hand to have variety throughout the week for your meals and snacks.

5. Spend a bit of time making a weekly meal plan so you can adjust your grocery list according to what you plan on making for the week. Then, spend an hour or two on a Sunday, or whatever day you want to dedicate, washing your fruits and veggies; making a chilli, soup, or other meal that you can make an extra batch of to freeze and take for lunches throughout the week. This can also be done with bars and cookies as well.

6. Making delicious, appealing recipes doesn't have to be complicated. Most of the recipes are easy and quick to make so you won't have to spend an entire day in the kitchen attempting to make a six-course meal. Unless, of course, that is what you enjoy doing.

BREAKFAST

Breakfast truly is the most important meal of the day. A great breakfast with a good serving of protein, healthy fats, and fruits and veggies sets the stage for more stable blood sugar, sustained energy, and an elevated mood.

When we are fueled optimally we are better able to carry out our day more productively at work, have a better workout, and less chances of having intense cravings for sugars and other refined foods. Whether your preference is a quick nutrient-packed smoothie or a savory egg-style dish, there are a few delicious options for everyone!

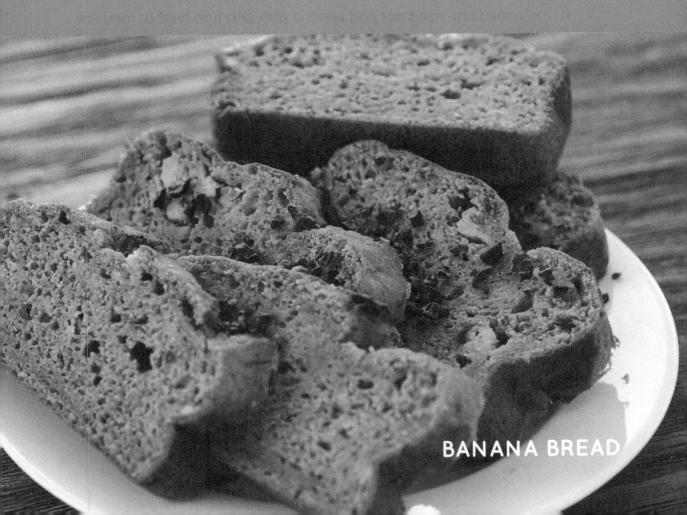

BANANA BREAD

APPLE CINNAMON QUINOA OATMEAL

Ingredients

2 medium-sized organic gala apples, chopped into small chunks or shredded

1 cup quinoa flakes

Tbsp. cinnamon

Handful of pecans or walnuts

1 tsp. maple syrup

1 ⅓ cups unsweetened almond milk

Method

1. In a medium-sized pot add almond milk and turn heat to medium.

2. Once milk is boiling, add quinoa flakes, cover with a lid, turn off heat and let sit 1-2 minutes to set and serve.

3. Add quinoa, apples, cinnamon, nuts, and maple syrup to a bowl, mix and serve!

    Depending on your love for cinnamon, you may find you want to add more or less. Also, feel free to add different nuts, seeds or nut butter to this recipe.

Prep Time 20 minutes   **Cook Time** 5 minutes   **Serves** 2-3

AVOCADO BLUEBERRY CHIA SMOOTHIE

Ingredients

½ a ripe avocado, pit removed

1 cup frozen blueberries

Handful of fresh raspberries

½ ripe banana

1 Tbsp. chia seeds

1 ½ cups unsweetened Coconut Almond Milk

2 medium leaves of black kale, ripped off stems

1 scoop plant-based protein (optional)

Method:

1. Wash raspberries and kale and scoop avocado out of shell.

2. Add all ingredients to a high-powered blender or food processor and blend until smooth and creamy.

    Adjust amount of milk for thickness, depending on preference.

    For protein powder, look for one with no artificial colors or flavours, ideally with stevia as the only sweetener. Some great brands include Vega & Sun Warrior.

Prep Time 10 minutes   Serves 1-2

BANANA BREAD FRENCH TOAST

Ingredients (For banana bread)

2 cups all-purpose gluten-free flour blend

2 tsp. baking powder

Pinch sea salt

1 Tbsp. cinnamon

½ cup applesauce

3 eggs

1 Tbsp. pure vanilla extract

7 ripe bananas

2 Tbsp. lucuma powder

¾ cup olive oil

½ tsp. ground chia

½ tsp. ground flax meal mixture

2 tsp. boiling water

Ingredients (For French toast)

1 banana, sliced

Dark grade maple syrup

3 eggs, beaten

2 tsp. cinnamon

Pinch sea salt

1 tsp. coconut oil

Method

1. Pre-heat oven to 375 degrees Fahrenheit.

2. Grease 2 medium-sized loaf pans with coconut oil.

3. In a large bowl combine flour, baking powder, cinnamon, lucuma powder & sea salt.

4. In a second bowl mash bananas then add applesauce, eggs, vanilla, and olive oil. Mix well.

5. In a small bowl add chia and flax meal to 2 tsp. boiling water and mix into a paste. Add to wet ingredients.

6. Combine dry and wet ingredients and pour into loaf pans. Bake for 40 minutes, check that a toothpick comes out clean in the center.

7. Remove loaves and place on a cooling rack.

8. Once cooled, slice loaves into 1-inch thick pieces.

9. Heat frying pan over medium heat and add coconut oil.

10. In a small bowl combine 3 eggs, cinnamon, and sea salt. Mix well.

11. Dip banana bread into egg mixture and add to frying pan. Cook until golden on both sides and serve with sliced banana, maple syrup, or coconut butter!

Prep Time 20 minutes   **Bake Time** 40 minutes
Frying French Toast 5 minutes   **Makes** 8-10 servings

CACAO AVOCADO SMOOTHIE

Ingredients

½ a ripe avocado, pit removed

1 ½ cups frozen berry mix with blueberry, raspberry, and strawberries

1 Tbsp. raw cacao powder

1 tsp. pure vanilla extract

½ ripe banana

1 Tbsp. chia seeds

1 ½ cups unsweetened flax milk

1 cup spinach leaves, rinsed

Method

1. Wash spinach and scoop avocado out of shell.
2. Add all ingredients to a high-powered blender or food processor and blend until smooth and creamy.
3. Adjust milk to desired consistency.

    If you are a huge chocolate fan, feel free to add extra raw cacao powder. It's full of antioxidants and magnesium.

***

Prep Time 10 minutes   **Serves** 1-2

CACAO RASPBERRY HEMP SMOOTHIE

Ingredients

2 Tbsp. hemp seeds

1 ½ cups frozen raspberries & strawberries

1 Tbsp. raw cacao powder

1 tsp. pure vanilla extract

½ ripe banana

1 Tbsp. chia seeds

1 ½ cups unsweetened coconut milk

1 cup kale leaves, pulled off stems

1 scoop plant-based protein (optional)

Method:

1. Wash kale and pull off stems.
2. Add all ingredients to a high-powered blender or food processor and blend until smooth and creamy.
3. Add extra milk for desired consistency.

Prep Time 10 minutes   **Serves** 1-2

FRENCH TOAST OMELETTE

Ingredients

3 medium-sized free-range or organic eggs

½ cup organic egg whites

Pinch sea salt

½ cup blueberries

½ cup raspberries

3 tsp. cinnamon

1 tsp. coconut oil

1 Tbsp. dark grade maple syrup

Method

1. Heat frying pan over medium/high heat and add coconut oil.
2. In a medium-sized bowl whisk eggs, egg white, sea salt, 1 ½ tsp. cinnamon together.
3. In a small bowl smash raspberries, blueberries and mix in other 1 ½ tsp. of cinnamon.
4. Add egg mixture to frying pan and cook on one side until golden and then flip omelette.
5. While omelette is cooking on second side, spread berry mixture over half the omelette and fold over once cooked.
6. Drizzle with dark grade maple syrup, sprinkle with more cinnamon and enjoy!

Prep Time 10 minutes   Cook Time 5-7 minutes   Serves 1-2

LUCUMA MAPLE NUT OATMEAL

Ingredients

½ cup quick- cooking gluten-free only oats

1 cup filtered water

Pinch sea salt

1 cup blueberries

1 tbspTbsp. almond butter

Handful of walnuts

2 tsp. cinnamon

1 tsp. lucuma powder

2tsp. maple syrup

2 tsp. hemp seeds

½ cup unsweetened almond milk

Method:

1. In a medium-sized pot add oats, water, and sea salt. Bring to a boil and then let simmer for about 3-5 minutes and stir occasionally until desired consistency is reached.

2. In a bowl, add all remaining ingredients to oatmeal and serve.

Prep Time 5 minutes   **Cook Time** 3-5 minutes   **Serves** 1-2

SAUTÉED ZUCCHINI BOWL WITH ROSEMARY GROUND TURKEY & SAUERKRAUT

Ingredients

1 medium-sized zucchini, chopped into cubes

1 yellow onion, diced

Handful of fresh dill, chopped

3 large leaves of rainbow or red chard, chopped

1 lb. lean ground turkey

Pinch of Himalayan sea salt

Pinch of garlic powder

Pinch of rosemary

Pinch of thyme

Pinch of black pepper

Pinch of basil

2 Tbsp. coconut oil

2 Tbsp. sauerkraut

Method

1. Place medium-sized frying pan over medium heat and melt 1 tsp. coconut oil.

2. In a second medium-sized frying pan melt other tsp. of coconut oil over medium heat.

3. Add ½ the diced yellow onion to each of the pans and sprinkle with sea salt and pepper. Stir occasionally until they are slightly caramelized.

4. Once the onions look golden, add the lean ground turkey to one pan with rosemary, thyme, basil, garlic, and sea salt then cook about 15-20 minutes, or until you break a piece of turkey open and it's white on the inside.

5. In the second pan, add zucchini, chard, and dill, stirring occasionally until vegetables are soft.

6. Combine turkey and vegetable mixture and stir well. Top with sauerkraut and adjust spices to taste.

Prep Time 10 minutes   **Cook Time** 15-20 minutes   Serves 2

STRAWBERRY BANANA BASIL SMOOTHIE

Ingredients

2 Tbsp. chia seeds

1 ½ cups frozen strawberries

3-5 fresh basil leaves

1 tsp. pure vanilla extract

½ ripe banana

1 ½ cups unsweetened brown rice milk

1 cup spinach leaves, washed

1 scoop plant-based protein (optional)

Method

1. Wash spinach leaves.
2. Add all ingredients to a high-powered blender or food processor and blend until smooth and creamy.
3. Add extra milk for desired consistency.

Prep Time 5 minutes   Serves 1-2

THE RADDEST PANCAKES

Ingredients

1 organic or free-range egg

1 cup unsweetened flax milk

1 ½ cups all-purpose gluten-free flour

Pinch sea salt

2 tsp. olive oil

1 tsp. coconut oil

1 Tbsp. baking powder

2 tsp. lucuma powder

1 tsp. pure vanilla extract

Maple syrup

Cinnamon

Bananas, blueberries, raspberries, or fruit of choice

Method

1. Heat frying pan to medium heat and melt coconut oil.

2. In a medium-sized bowl combine flour, sea salt, baking powder, lucuma powder, and sea salt.

3. In another bowl combine egg, olive oil, milk, and vanilla. Mix well.

4. Whisk wet ingredients into dry and adjust thickness of batter to your preference. You may need to add an extra tsp. or 2 of flour to get it perfect.

5. Pour batter into pan, flip once bubbles appear on top of the pancake and the underside is golden brown.

6. Once both sides are golden, serve with coconut butter, maple syrup, fruit, or cinnamon.

Prep Time 10 minutes   **Makes** 6-8 pancakes

VEGGIE OMELETTE

Ingredients (For the Omelette)

1 tsp. coconut oil

3 organic or free-range eggs

½ cup organic egg whites

Few sprigs freshly chopped dill

3-4 fresh basil leaves, chopped, or 1 tsp. of dried basil

Pinch of garlic powder

Pinch of Himalayan sea salt

Pinch of black pepper

Cilantro to garnish

Ingredients (For sautéed veggies)

½ yellow onion, diced

½ bell pepper, diced (red, yellow, orange)

½ zucchini, diced

2 cups fresh greens of choice (chard, spinach, spring mix)

Handful of chopped dill

Method

1. With a fork, whisk eggs in a bowl then add spices and dill.
2. Heat a medium-sized frying pan over medium heat and add coconut oil.
3. Have a second pan ready for the egg mixture to make the omelet.
4. Add yellow onion, garlic, sea salt, pepper, and dill to the coconut oil in heated pan.
5. Once the onions have been sautéed for a few minutes, add the rest of the vegetables, spices, and greens.
6. Add the coconut milk to the vegetables and cover with a lid, stirring occasionally for 10-15 minutes, depending how crisp or cooked you like your veggies.
7. Right before the veggies are cooked to your liking, heat coconut oil in the other pan over medium-high heat.
8. Add the egg mixture so it evenly spreads throughout whole pan.
9. Flip omelet once golden brown on the bottom, then add sautéed veggies to one half, garnish with cilantro.

Prep Time 10 minutes   **Cook Time** 15-20 minutes   **Serves** 2

YAM HASH & BASIL ROSEMARY TURKEY BOWL

Ingredients

1 medium-sized yam, shredded

1 yellow onion, diced

Handful of fresh dill, chopped

1 lb. lean ground turkey

Pinch of Himalayan sea salt

Pinch of garlic powder

Pinch of rosemary

Pinch of thyme

Pinch of black pepper

Pinch of basil

Pinch of cinnamon

2 Tbsp. coconut oil

Method

1. Heat medium-sized frying pan over medium heat and melt 1 tsp. coconut oil.

2. In a second medium-sized frying pan melt the other tsp. of coconut oil over medium heat.

3. Shred yam with a cheese grater and set aside.

4. Add ½ the diced yellow onion to each of the pans and sprinkle with sea salt and pepper. Stir occasionally until they appear caramelized.

5. Once the onions look golden, add the lean ground turkey to one pan with the rosemary, thyme, basil, garlic, and sea salt. Cook about 15-20 minutes, or until you break a piece of turkey open and it's white on the inside.

6. In the second pan, after coconut oil is heated, add shredded yams, sea salt, pepper, cinnamon, and basil, stirring occasionally until yam pieces are soft.

7. Combine turkey and yam mixture. Stir well and enjoy.

Prep Time 10 minutes   Cook Time 20-25 minutes   Serves 3-4

DIPS & DRESSINGS

I found that a lot of the dips and dressings I used to eat were full of hydrogenated oils, MSG, sugar, poor-quality dairy, and other ingredients that wreaked havoc on my stomach. I wanted to create some of my favourites, in a more healthy way, then add in something different that is tasty and satisfying. These can be put on crackers or paleo burgers, spread into omelets, served with raw or roasted veggies. I enjoy experimenting with cashews, which are one of my new favourites to make dips and icings with. They give a creamy texture and a nice taste.

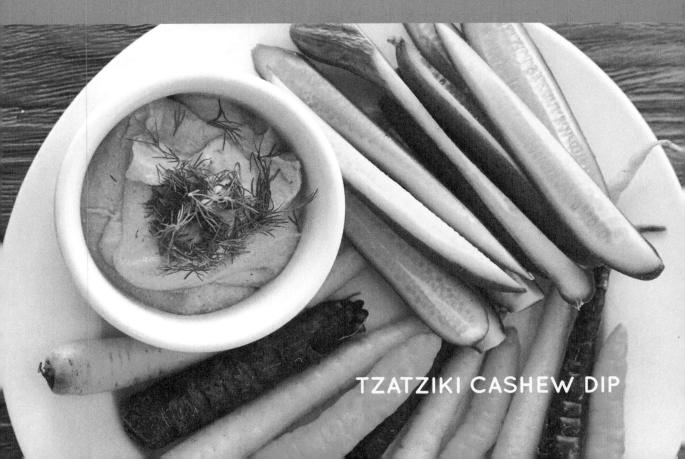

TZATZIKI CASHEW DIP

EASIEST GUACAMOLE

Ingredients

3 medium-sized ripe avocados, scooped out of the shell

2 cloves garlic, finely chopped

2 tsp. freshly squeezed lemon or lime

Pinch Himalayan sea salt

Pinch garlic powder

Pinch chilli powder

Pinch black pepper

Method

1. Remove pits from avocados and scoop out of shell into a bowl.
2. Mash and add in all remaining ingredients.
3. Adjust lemon and spices to taste.

Prep Time 5 minutes   **Makes** about 1 cup of guacamole

COCONUT HERB SPREAD

Ingredients

½ cup coconut oil, softened

Pinch of sea salt

Pinch of black pepper

Pinch of garlic powder

Pinch of basil

Pinch of rosemary

Method

1. Add coconut oil to bowl and mash with a fork to soften.
2. Add spices and mix well.
3. Use on roasted or steamed veggies, in mashed potatoes or yams, or as a spread on savoury muffins, breads or crackers.

Prep Time 5 minutes   **Makes** about ½ cup of spread

CURRY CASHEW DIP

Ingredients

1 cup soaked raw cashews

Pinch sea salt

Pinch garlic powder

1 tsp. madras curry powder

¼ cup olive oil

Method

1. Soak cashews in filtered water, with a pinch of sea salt, for at least 20-30 minutes.

2. Rinse cashews and add all ingredients to a high-powered blender or food processor and blend until creamy.

3. Adjust flavour to your liking. Some people prefer a slight curry taste whereas others prefer a very strong, spicy flavour.

Prep Time 5 minutes   **Makes** about 1 ½ cups of dip   **Keeps** in the fridge 3-4 days

GARLIC CASHEW DIP

Ingredients

1 cup soaked raw cashews

Pinch sea salt

Pinch garlic powder

3 roasted garlic cloves

¼ cup olive oil

1 tsp. lucuma powder

Squeeze of fresh lemon

Method

1. Soak cashews in filtered water, with a pinch of sea salt, for at least 20-30 minutes.

2. Rinse cashews and add all ingredients to a high-powered blender or food processor and blend until creamy.

3. Use spices to adjust flavour to your liking. If you want a more tangy dip add more lemon.

Prep Time 5 minutes   **Makes** about 1 ½ cups of dip   **Keeps** in the fridge 3-4 days

ROSEMARY TURKEY GRAVY

Ingredients

½ cup gluten-free all-purpose flour

½ cup filtered water

2 cups turkey drippings

2 tsp. Himalayan sea salt

2 tsp. black pepper

2 tsp. garlic powder

2 cups potato water

Method

1. Pour potato water into medium-sized pot and bring to boil over medium heat.

2. Combine spices, flour, and filtered water in a bowl, then whisk until no clumps of flour remain.

3. Add the flour mixture and turkey drippings to the potato water, then whisk thoroughly.

4. Simmer and stir until desired consistency is reached, keeping at low heat to serve.

Prep Time 5 minutes   **Makes** about 2 cups of dip   **Keeps** in the fridge 3-4 days

ROASTED RED PEPPER CASHEW DIP

Ingredients (For the roasted veggies)

2 red bell peppers

3 cloves garlic, finely chopped

½ yellow onion, chopped

2 Tbsp. coconut oil

1 tsp. sea salt

Pinch of oregano

Pinch of garlic powder

Pinch of black pepper

Pinch of rosemary

Ingredients (For the dip)

1 cup raw cashews, soaked in filtered water

Pinch sea salt

1 tsp. garlic powder

¼ cup olive oil

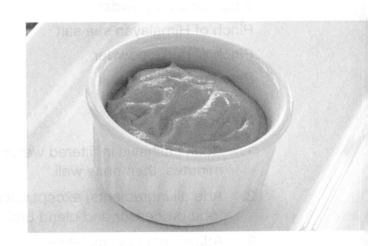

Method

1. 1. Heat oven to 375 degrees Fahrenheit.

2. Slice peppers in half and clean out seeds. Chop into long slices and add to an oven-proof baking dish.

3. Chop onion and garlic and add to peppers, along with spices and coconut oil, then mix well with hands.

4. In the meantime, soak cashews in filtered water with a pinch of sea salt for 20-30 minutes. Rinse well.

5. Roast in the oven for about 25-30 minutes, until the peppers are soft.

6. Add roasted peppers, cashews, sea salt, garlic powder, and olive oil to high-speed blender or food processor and mix until creamy. Adjust to desired flavour.

Prep Time 10 minutes   **Cook Time** 30 minutes   **Makes** about 1 ½ cups of dip

Goes great with the Paleo burgers or veggie sticks   **Keeps** in the fridge 3-4 days

For a **more tangy version** add a tablespoon of apple cider vinegar

TZATZIKI CASHEW DIP

Ingredients

1 ¼ cups raw cashews, soaked in filtered water

3 mini cucumbers, chopped into small pieces

Handful of dill, chopped

½ fresh lemon, squeezed

¼ cup olive oil

1 tsp. lucuma powder

Pinch of Himalayan sea salt

Pinch of garlic powder

Pinch of black pepper

Method

1. Soak cashews in filtered water, with a pinch of sea salt, for 20-30 minutes, then rinse well.

2. Add all ingredients, except cucumbers, to high-powered blender or food processor and blend until creamy.

3. Adjust taste to your liking—I like extra garlic and dill in mine.

4. Mix in cucumber and serve.

Prep Time 5 minutes   **Makes** about 4 ½ cups of gravy

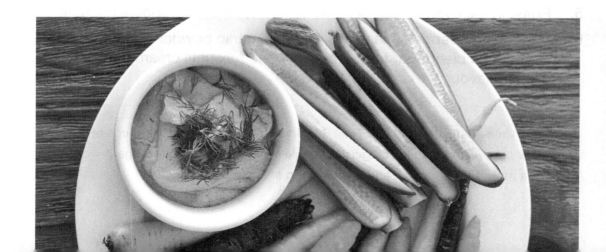

SIDE DISHES, SALADS, SOUPS & ENTREES

Side dishes, salads, soups, and entrees are easy to make larger portions of ahead of time so you can have it prepared for throughout the week. This is especially nice when you are on the run. Instead of making poor food choices you can grab some soup from the freezer, or pile some pre-made salad into a container. This way you can get to where you need to be without sacrificing healthy eating. Have fun experimenting with salads and savory side dishes by using different spices and oils.

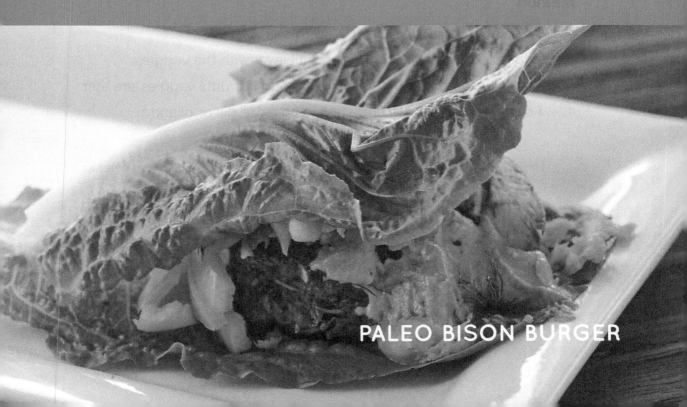

PALEO BISON BURGER

BEET VEGGIE SOUP

Ingredients

5 large carrots, diced

5 stocks celery, diced

1 medium-sized zucchini, diced

1 medium-sized yellow onion, diced

4 medium-sized red or yellow beets, chopped into small cubes

1 cup dill, finely chopped

2 tsp. Himalayan sea salt

Pinch of pepper

Pinch of thyme

Pinch of garlic

Pinch of rosemary

7-8 cups of filtered water

Method

1. Wash and chop all veggies. Add to a crockpot.
2. Add spices, then fill with water until level with the veggies.
3. Turn on low heat and cook for 5-6 hours, or until veggies are soft.
4. Adjust spices to taste and serve with extra dill or cilantro.

Prep Time 20 minutes   **Cook Time** 5-6 hours   **Makes** 5-6 services of soup

BASIC BONE BROTH

Ingredients

2-3 large organic beef bones
Squeeze of fresh lemon

Method

1. Set oven to 350 degrees Fahrenheit.

2. Put bones on a cookie sheet and squeeze lemon on them to help release mineral availability.

3. Bake for 30 minutes if thawed, or about 60 minutes if bones are frozen.

4. Take bones out of oven and add to a boiling pot of water or a slow cooker on high heat.

5. After about 10-20 minutes, scoop foam off the top and continue to simmer for at least 24 hours, adding a bit of extra water if the level gets low.

6. Drink on its own to help support strengthening the intestinal lining, or add as a broth to other soups.

Prep Time 20 minutes   **Cook Time** 24 hours   **Makes** 7-8 cups of broth

BISON & QUINOA STUFFED PEPPERS

Ingredients

1 yellow onion, diced

1 lb. lean ground organic or grass-finished bison

4 medium chard leaves, chopped into small pieces

4 whole red bell peppers with the stem and seeds scooped out

1 cup quinoa

2 cups filtered water

Large handful of dill, chopped finely

3 Tbsp. coconut oil

2 cloves garlic, finely chopped

Pinch Himalayan sea salt

Pinch pepper

Pinch garlic powder

Pinch oregano

Pinch rosemary

Method

1. Pre-heat oven to 350 degrees Fahrenheit.

2. Heat 1 Tbsp. coconut oil in frying pan, over medium heat.

3. Add onion, sea salt, and pepper, then sauté until onions are slightly caramelized.

4. Add bison, sea salt, pepper, garlic powder, rosemary, basil, and oregano. Stir well until bison is brown almost all the way through.

5. Bring 1 cup of water and a pinch of sea salt to a boil in a medium-sized pot. Add quinoa and turn to low heat, then cover for about 15 minutes.

6. Meanwhile, wash peppers then chop the tops off, scooping out the seeds.

7. Finely chop dill and chard, then set aside.

8. Once the quinoa and bison are cooked, mix them together with chard, dill, spices, and 1 Tbsp. coconut oil. Fill the peppers.

9. Place stuffed peppers in an oven-proof baking dish and bake for about 30-40 minutes until bison has completely browned.

Prep Time 15 minutes   Cook Time 55-75 minutes   Serves 4

CHEWY ROASTED VEGGIE CHIPS (2 WAYS)

Ingredients (for Sea Salt & Pepper Chips)

1 large yam, cut into thin chip slices about ½ cm thick

1 large sweet potato, sliced into ½ cm thick pieces

3 Tbsp. olive oil

Pinch Himalayan sea salt to taste

Pinch black pepper to taste

Ingredients (for Sea Salt & Pepper Chips)

1 large yam, cut into thin chip slices about ½ cm thick

1 large sweet potato, sliced into ½ cm thick pieces

3 Tbsp. olive oil

Pinch Himalayan sea salt to taste

1 handful fresh dill, chopped

Pinch garlic powder to taste

Method

1. Preheat oven to 350 degrees Fahrenheit.
2. Place parchment paper over two separate cookie sheets and cover with one layer of the veggie slices.
3. Add spices and olive oil then mix thoroughly with hands. Put in oven for about 60-90 minutes.
4. Halfway through baking, flip the chips over.

Prep Time 15 minutes Cook Time 60-90 minutes Serves 4-5

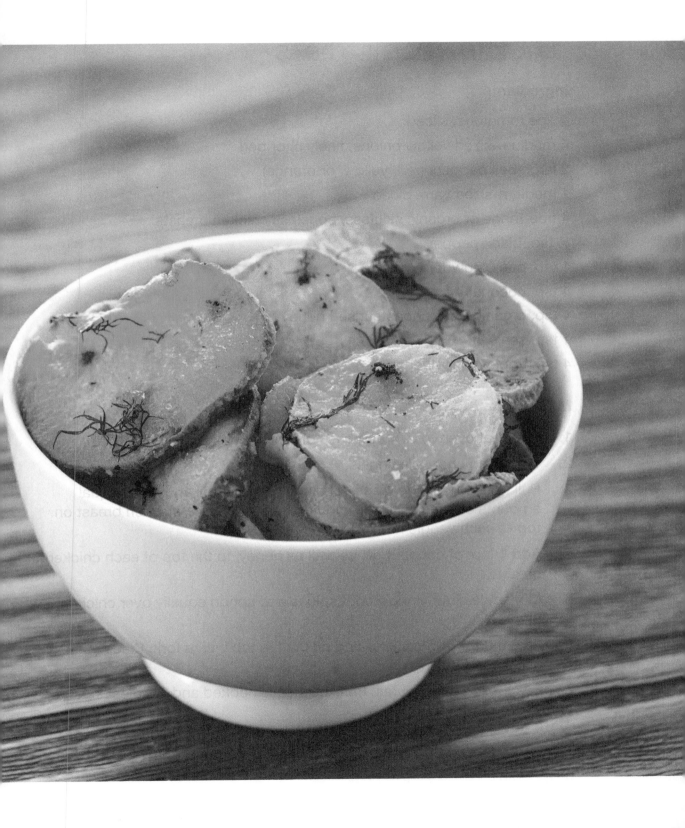

CHICKEN VEGGIE NESTS

Ingredients

4 ripe tomatoes, sliced

4 medium-sized yellow onions, finely chopped

2 large bell peppers (red, yellow, or orange)

1 medium-sized yam, diced

4 free-range or organic skinless, boneless chicken breasts

½ tsp. black pepper

1 tsp. garlic powder

4 tsp. coconut oil

4 tsp. organic, raw, unpasteurised honey

1 tsp. sea salt

4 tsp. apple cider vinegar

Method

1. Pre-heat oven to 375 degrees Fahrenheit.
2. Wash and chop all veggies.
3. Pull and tear 4 large pieces of aluminum-free foil and place equal amounts of veggies in the middle of each. Place a chicken breast on top of each veggie nest.
4. Add 1 tsp. of coconut oil, as well as honey, to the top of each chicken breast.
5. Mix apple cider vinegar with spices and spoon equally over chicken breasts.
6. Fold the foil into packets and pierce the top with a fork. Place in an oven-proof baking dish.
7. Bake for 35-40 minutes, until chicken is cooked and veggies are soft.

Prep Time 20 minutes   **Cook Time** 35-40 minutes   **Serves** 4

CREAMY DILL SWEET POTATOES

Ingredients

1 medium-sized sweet potato, chopped into small cubes

1 yellow onion, diced

Large handful of dill, chopped finely

1 Tbsp. coconut oil

2 cloves garlic, finely chopped

2 ½ to 3 cups unsweetened coconut milk

Pinch Himalayan sea salt

Pinch pepper

Pinch garlic powder

Method

1.   Melt coconut oil in a medium-sized pot, over medium heat.

2.   Add onion, dill, and spices. Stir well.

3.   Add coconut milk and simmer for 25-30 minutes, until sweet potato is soft.

Prep Time 10 minutes   **Cook Time** 25-30 minutes   **Serves** 3-4

SIDE DISHES, SALADS, SOUPS & ENTREES

EGG SALAD ROLLS

Ingredients

6 eggs, boiled

Half a cup chopped green onions

5-6 large romaine, or green leaf, lettuce washed

1 large carrot, grated

2 mini cucumbers, grated

1 ripe avocado with pit removed

Handful of chopped dill

1 ½ Tbsp. apple cider vinegar

Pinch Himalayan sea salt

Pinch of black pepper

Pinch of garlic powder

Method

1. In a medium-sized pot, boil water and drop in eggs to cook for 20 minutes.

2. After eggs are boiled and cooled, peel and add them to a bowl with avocado, apple cider vinegar, spices, and dill. Mash until mixture is well combined.

3. Wash the lettuce leaves and pat them dry with paper towel.

4. Evenly spread the egg mixture on the lettuce and top with carrot, cucumber, and green onion. Roll the wraps closed.

Prep Time 25 minutes   **Cook Time** 20 minutes   **Serves** 5-6

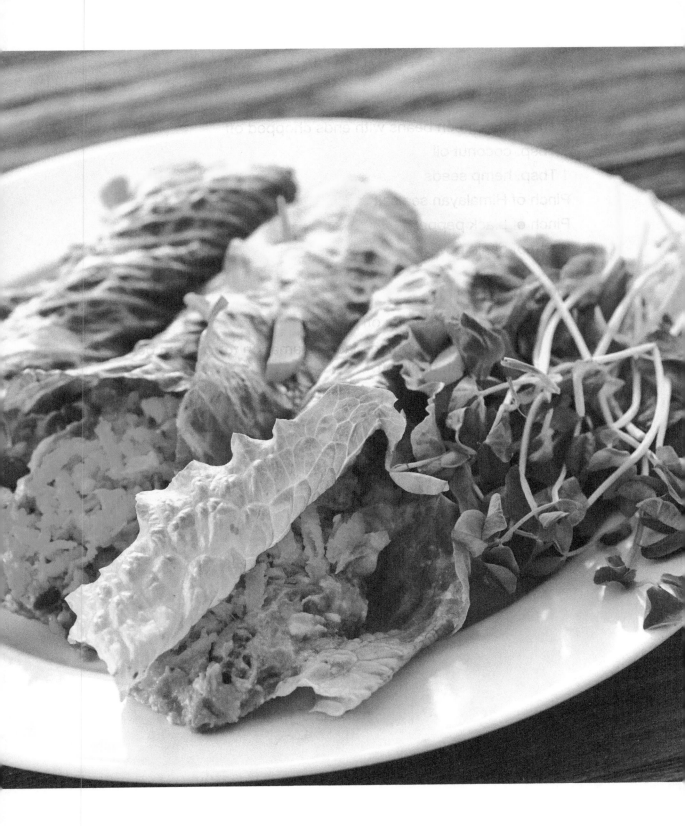

GARLIC GREEN BEANS

Ingredients

3 cups fresh green beans with ends chopped off

1 Tbsp. coconut oil

1 Tbsp. hemp seeds

Pinch of Himalayan sea salt

Pinch of black pepper

Pinch of garlic powder

Method

1. Wash and pinch ends off beans.

2. Add water to a pot then place steamer on top. Steam beans over medium heat, until soft.

3. Add steamed green beans, spices, coconut oil, and hemp seeds to a bowl. Mix well and serve.

Prep Time 10 minutes   **Cook Time** 20 minutes   **Serves** 3-4

GARLIC & DILL SMASHED POTATOES

Ingredients

4-5 medium-sized potatoes, peeled and cut into quarters

2 Tbsp. coconut oil

3 Tbsp. unsweetened coconut milk

Pinch of Himalayan sea salt

Pinch of black pepper

Pinch of garlic powder

3 cloves of garlic, crushed

Handful of fresh dill, chopped

Method

1. Add a pinch of sea salt to a medium-sized pot of water and bring to a boil.

2. Add potatoes and garlic cloves, then continue to boil until potatoes are soft—about 20-25 minutes.

3. Drain water, add coconut oil, spices, and coconut milk, then mash with a potato masher until desired consistency is reached. It can be chunky or creamy; it's up to you.

Prep Time 10 minutes   **Cook Time** 20-25 minutes   **Serves** 3-4

GARAM MASALA BUTTERNUT SQUASH SOUP

Ingredients

1 medium-sized butternut squash, peeled and cut into cubes

1 large yellow onion, finely chopped

3 cloves garlic, finely chopped

2 cups unsweetened coconut milk

1 ½ cups filtered water

Large handful of dill, chopped

1 Tbsp. cinnamon

2 Tbsp. garam masala spice

2 Tbsp. coconut oil

Pinch Himalayan sea salt

Pinch of black pepper

Method

1. Put a large pot on medium heat.

2. Add onion, garlic, dill, sea salt, pepper, and coconut oil then sauté until onions appear caramelized.

3. Add butternut squash, cinnamon, garam masala, coconut milk, and water. Cover and simmer over medium heat, stirring occasionally for about 25-30 minutes, until squash is soft.

4. Once squash is cooked, pour entire contents into a high-speed blender or food processor and blend until creamy and smooth.

5. Adjust spices to taste and top with dill.

Prep Time 15 minutes   **Cook Time** 25-30 minutes   Serves 4-5

OVEN ROASTED YAM FRIES

Ingredients

1 large yam

2 Tbsp. coconut oil

Handful of dill, chopped finely

Pinch of cinnamon

Pinch of Himalayan sea salt

Pinch of black pepper

Pinch of oregano

Pinch of rosemary

Method

1. Pre-heat oven to 350 degrees Fahrenheit.
2. Slice yam into fry-size pieces and place on a cookie sheet lined with parchment paper.
3. Add spices, dill, and coconut oil. Mix thoroughly.
4. Bake in the oven for 30-35 minutes, or until soft.

Prep Time 10 minutes   **Cook Time** 30-35 minutes   **Serves** 3-4

OVEN ROASTED BEETS

Ingredients

4 large beets, chopped into small cubes

1 yellow onion, finely chopped

Large handful of dill, finely chopped

2 cloves garlic, finely chopped

3 Tbsp. coconut oil

1 tsp. rosemary

1 tsp. Himalayan sea salt

1 tsp. black pepper

1 tsp. garlic powder

Method

1. Pre-heat oven to 375 degrees Fahrenheit.
2. Wash beets and then chop with onion, garlic, and dill. Add to an oven-proof baking dish.
3. Add coconut oil and spices to beets then mix thoroughly.
4. Roast in the oven for 25-30 minutes or until beets are soft.

Prep Time 15 minutes   **Cook Time** 25-30 minutes   **Serves** 4-5

PALEO BISON OR TURKEY BURGERS

Ingredients

1 lb. lean ground bison or turkey

½ yellow onion, finely chopped

2 gloves garlic, finely chopped

Handful of fresh dill, chopped

1 egg

1 tsp. coconut oil

Pinch of Himalayan sea salt

Pinch of rosemary

Pinch of sage

Pinch of garlic powder

Pinch of basil

Pinch of black pepper

10 large romaine or green-leaf lettuce leaves

1 ripe avocado, pit removed and sliced

½ long English cucumber, thinly sliced

Package of pea shoots

½ lemon, squeezed

Method

1. Combine meat, spices, egg, onion, and garlic in a bowl and mix thoroughly with hands. Shape into medium-sized patties.

2. Heat a frying pan on medium and add coconut oil.

3. Add patties to pan and flip after about 6-8 minutes, once underside is brown.

4. Cover with a lid to keep the meat moist and flip again after another 6-8 minutes, once the other side is nice and brown. Check occasionally so they don't overcook.

5. Pierce one through the middle with a knife to make sure it's brown all the way through.

6. Add burgers to lettuce with avocado, cucumber, and pea shoots. Distribute lemon over top and enjoy.

Prep Time 15-20 minutes   **Cook Time** 16-20 minutes   **Serves** 5-6

I also recommend serving the Tzatziki or Roasted Red Pepper Dip on these!

RAD RAINBOW SALAD

Ingredients

5 cups spring mix salad

Handful of fresh dill, finely chopped

Handful of cilantro, chopped

2 red beets, shredded

3 large carrots, shredded

1 yellow bell pepper, finely chopped

6 large strawberries, finely chopped

½ cup pumpkin seeds

1 cup purple cabbage, finely chopped

½ cup chives, finely chopped

1 cup blueberries

½ cup hemp seeds

1 long English cucumber, chopped into cubes

½ cup apple cider vinegar

3 Tbsp. avocado or flax seed oil

Pinch of Himalayan sea salt

Pinch of black pepper

Pinch of oregano

Pinch of garlic powder

Pinch of chilli powder

Method

1.   1. Wash spring mix and add to a large bowl.

2.   Shred carrot and beet and add to spring mix.

3.   Chop and wash all vegetables and add to spring mix.

4.   Sprinkle hemp seeds, pumpkin seeds, strawberries, blueberries, dill, chives, and cilantro over veggie salad.

5. In a jar, add spices, apple cider vinegar, and oil of choice. Shake well.

6. Pour dressing over salad and toss lightly.

Prep Time 20 minutes   **Serves** 3-4

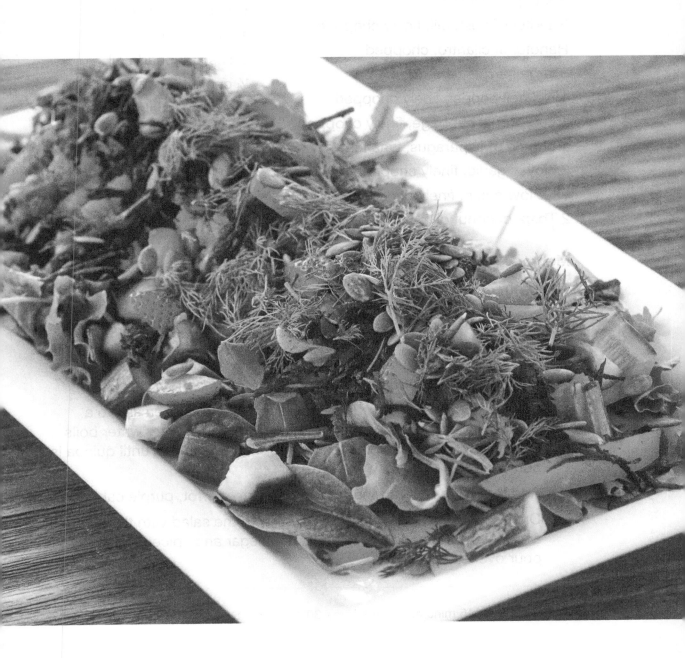

ROASTED ASPARAGUS & RED PEPPER QUINOA SALAD

Ingredients

3-4 cups spring mix
Handful of fresh dill, finely chopped
Handful of cilantro, chopped
3 large carrots, shredded
1 red bell pepper, finely chopped
1 cup purple cabbage, finely chopped
1 bundle of asparagus, washed
2 cloves garlic, finely chopped
½ yellow onion, finely chopped
2 Tbsp. coconut oil

½ cup white quinoa
1 cup filtered water
3 Tbsp. avocado oil
¼ cup apple cider vinegar
Pinch of Himalayan sea salt
Pinch of black pepper
Pinch of oregano
Pinch of garlic powder
Pinch of chilli powder

Method

1. Pre-heat oven to 350 degrees Fahrenheit.
2. Wash asparagus and red bell pepper.
3. Place parchment on a cookie sheet and add onion, asparagus, garlic, bell pepper, coconut oil, black pepper and sea salt and bake in the oven for about 20-25 minutes until veggies are soft.
4. In the meantime, add 1 cup of water and a pinch of sea salt to a medium pot set on high heat until water is boiling. After water boils add quinoa and cook at low heat for about 15 minutes until quinoa is cooked.
5. Add to a large bowl spring mix, dill, cilantro, carrot, purple cabbage.
6. Once the veggies are cooked add them to the salad with the quinoa and mix the avocado oil, apple cider vinegar and spices in a jar and pour over salad. Enjoy!

Prep Time 15 minutes   **Cook Time** 30 minutes   Serves 3-4

SHEPHERD'S PIE

Ingredients

1 lb. lean ground white turkey

1 yellow onion, finely chopped

Handful of dill, chopped

5 medium-sized carrots, finely chopped

1 cup peas, fresh or frozen

2 cups green beans, finely chopped

1 large yam, chopped into cubes

3 Tbsp. coconut oil

1 cup unsweetened coconut milk

2 Tbsp. arrowroot powder plus 2 Tbsp. water

4 Tbsp. basil

5 Tbsp. garlic powder

3 Tbsp. sea salt

Pinch of black pepper

4 Tbsp. rosemary

Method

1. Preheat oven to 350 degrees Fahrenheit.

2. In a large frying pan, over medium-high heat, add coconut oil, onion, dill, pinch of sea salt, and pepper. Sauté until onions are caramelized.

3. Add turkey and remainder of spices then cook until brown, about 15-20 minutes.

4. In the meantime, wash and chop yam then add to a steamer until soft.

5. Add chopped beans, carrots, and peas to the turkey once it's browned, then stir.

6. Measure arrowroot powder and cold water, then mix into a paste and pour over turkey and veggie mixture. Simmer for about 10 minutes.

7. Add the turkey-veggie mixture to an oven-proof baking dish.

8. After yams are cooked, mash them in a bowl and add 2 Tbsp. coconut oil, sea salt, pepper, and garlic powder to taste. Spread over the top of the veggie and turkey mixture.

9. Bake for 30-45 minutes, until carrots are cooked in the middle.

Prep Time 20 minutes   **Cook Time** 45-65 minutes   **Serves** 6-8

SMASHED YAMS

Ingredients

1 medium-sized yam, chopped into cubes

Handful of fresh dill, finely chopped

2 Tbsp. coconut oil

Pinch of Himalayan sea salt

Pinch of black pepper

Pinch of garlic powder

Pinch of cinnamon

Method

1. Wash, then chop yam into small cubes.

2. Fill a steaming pot with water and add yam to steamer for 20-25 minutes, until yams are soft.

3. Add cooked yams, dill, coconut oil, and spices to a bowl then mash into desired consistency.

Prep Time 10 minutes   **Cook Time** 20-25 minutes   **Serves** 3-4

SWEETS, TREATS & DESSERTS

One of the things I really wanted to work toward was creating some of my favourite baked goods and sweet treats in a more healthy way so the ingredients have more nutrient value and they don't impact blood sugar levels as much, or impact digestion in a negative way. Most of us like to enjoy something sweet now and again, so it's nice to have the options that will support that.

Getting through my sugar addiction was a huge struggle, but after I cut out the white stuff and started to use more natural sweeteners, I found I could enjoy my treats and not find myself wanting to eat the whole batch at once. Being satisfied makes me feel at peace, like I can enjoy my treat and then move on to the next part of my day, knowing that my body could benefit what I just gave it.

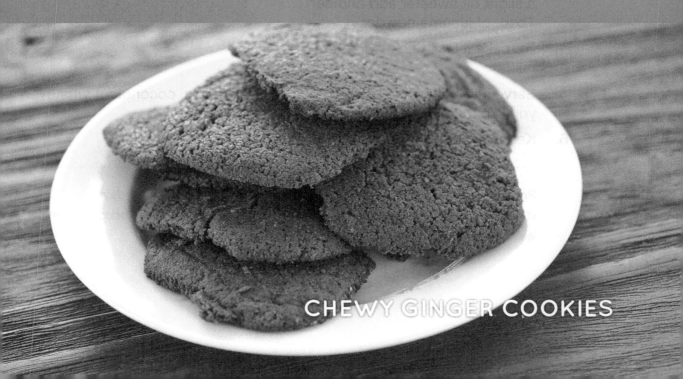

CHEWY GINGER COOKIES

AVOCADO CHOCOLATE PUDDING

Ingredients

4 ripe avocados

7 Tbsp. raw cacao powder

4-5 Tbsp. lucuma powder

1 Tbsp. organic vanilla extract

½ cup unsweetened coconut or almond milk

½ cup dark grade maple syrup

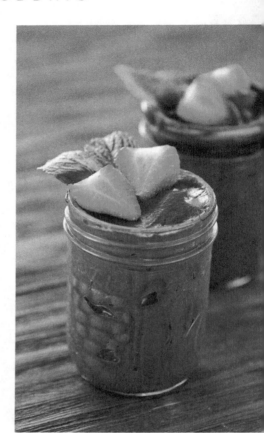

Method

1. Remove pit and shell from avocado.

2. Add all ingredients into a high-speed blender or food processer and blend until smooth and creamy.

3. Adjust flavour to taste, to make a slight bit sweeter add another Tbsp. of lucuma powder.

4. To make it less thick, add more milk.

5. Serve into bowls and top with berries, cacao nibs, coconut (or whatever you like.)

6. Keeps chilled in fridge for 2-3 days

Prep Time 10 minutes   **Serves** 4-5   **Keeps** chilled in fridge for 2-3 days

Garnish with raspberries, cacao nibs, chopped hazelnuts, shredded coconut or mint leaves

BAKED PEARS WITH CINNAMON CRUMBLE

Ingredients

4 ripe green pears

¾ cup walnuts or pecans (or a bit of both), crushed

½ cup raisins

¼ cup shredded unsweetened coconut

¼ cup coconut oil, softened or melted

2 tsp. coconut palm sugar

1 tsp. organic vanilla extract

1 Tbsp. cinnamon (add more if you love it)

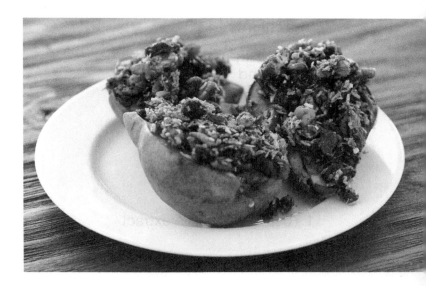

Method

1. Pre-heat oven to 375 degrees Fahrenheit.

2. Slice pears in half and scoop out the core to make room for the filling. Place in an oven-proof baking dish.

3. In a medium-sized bowl combine all of the ingredients and mix well until crumble is sticky.

4. Fill cored pears with crumble mixture and put in the oven for 17-20 minutes.

5. To check they are done, pierce the pears with a fork to ensure they are nice and soft.

6. Serve alone or with coconut ice cream or over gluten-free oatmeal or quinoa.

Prep Time 15 minutes   **Cook Time** 17-20 minutes   **Serves** 8

BANANA BREAD

Ingredients

2 cups all-purpose gluten-free flour blend

2 tsp. baking powder

Pinch sea salt

1 Tbsp. cinnamon

½ cup applesauce

3 eggs

1 Tbsp. pure vanilla extract

7 ripe bananas

2 Tbsp. lucuma powder

¾ cup olive oil

½ tsp. ground chia

½ tsp. ground flax meal mixture

2 tsp. boiling water

Method

1. Pre-heat oven to 375 degrees Fahrenheit.

2. Grease 2 medium-sized loaf pans with coconut oil.

3. In a large bowl combine flour, baking powder, cinnamon, lucuma powder, and sea salt.

4. In a second bowl, mash bananas and add applesauce, eggs, vanilla, and olive oil, then mix well.

5. In a small bowl, mix chia and flax meal with 2 tsp. boiling water and stir into a paste. Add to wet ingredients.

6. Combine dry and wet ingredients then pour into loaf pans and bake for 40 minutes. Check that a toothpick comes out clean from the center when done.

7. Remove loaves and place on a cooling rack.

8. Slice loaves into inch-thick pieces and enjoy.

Prep Time 15-20 minutes   **Bake Time** 40 minutes   **Makes** 2 medium sized loaves
Spread some coconut oil and a sprinkle of sea salt on a warm slice—it's divine!

DIVINE BANANA VANILLA SOFT SERVE

Ingredients

4 bananas out of the peel, frozen

5 Tbsp. cacao powder

1 tsp. pure vanilla extract

2 Tbsp. lucuma powder

2 Tbsp. maple syrup

1 cup unsweetened coconut milk

4 Tbsp. cacao nibs

½ cup hazelnut butter (optional)

Method

1. Peel 4 bananas and place in a Ziploc in the freezer until frozen

2. Add all ingredients, except cacao nibs, into a food processor or high-speed blender and blend until creamy and smooth.

3. Divide into bowls and top with cacao nibs.

Prep Time 5 minutes   **Serves** 4

Add hazelnut butter for a choco-hazelnut flavour—it's divine!

BASIC CHOCOLATE

Ingredients

3 cups cacao butter

1 cup coconut oil

6-8 Tbsp. raw cacao powder (depending how rich you like your chocolate)

¾ cup dark grade maple syrup

1 tsp. pure vanilla extract

1 tsp. maca powder

4 Tbsp. lucuma powder

Method

1. Add cacao butter to pot and stir over medium heat until melted.

2. Turn heat off and whisk in all other ingredients and mix well.

3. Add chocolate to molds, or place parchment into a square or rectangular shaped glass dish and pour chocolate evenly over parchment.

4. Put container in the freezer to set.

5. Break into chocolate bark pieces and enjoy.

Prep Time 5 minutes   **Cook Time** 10-15 minutes   **Makes** 16-24 medium sized chocolates

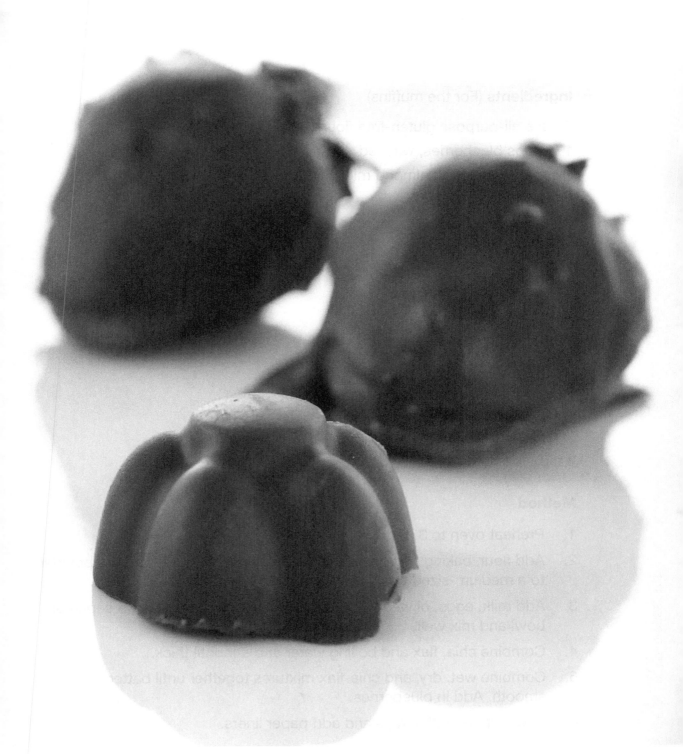

BURSTING BLUEBERRY MUFFINS WITH PECAN CRUMBLE

Ingredients (For the muffins)

2 cups all-purpose gluten-free flour

1 ½ cups blueberries, washed

1 cup unsweetened almond milk

2 tsp. baking powder

¾ cup raw, organic, unpasteurised honey

¾ cup olive oil

2 organic or free-range eggs

½ cup applesauce

½ cup hemp hearts

1 Tbsp. cinnamon

4 Tbsp. lucuma powder

½ tsp. ground chia

½ tsp. ground flax meal mixture

2 tsp. boiling water

Ingredients (For the cinnamon crumble)

½ cup coconut oil

1 cup ground pecans

1 tsp. sea salt

½ cup coconut sugar

1 Tbsp. cinnamon

Method

1. Preheat oven to 375 degrees Fahrenheit.
2. Add flour, baking powder, hemp hearts, cinnamon, and lucuma powder to a medium-sized bowl and mix.
3. Add milk, eggs, olive oil, honey, applesauce, and vanilla to a separate bowl and mix well.
4. Combine chia, flax and boiling water and stir until thick.
5. Combine wet, dry, and chia-flax mixtures together until batter is smooth. Add in blueberries.
6. Take 2 mini-muffin trays and add paper liners.

7. Spoon batter into muffin trays.

8. Combine all ingredients for cinnamon crumble into a bowl and mix well.

9. Spoon cinnamon mixture over the top of each muffin to cover surface.

10. Bake for about 25 minutes.

11. Test with a toothpick and when it comes out clean they are ready.

Prep Time 20 minutes   **Cook Time** 25 minutes   **Makes** 38 mini muffins

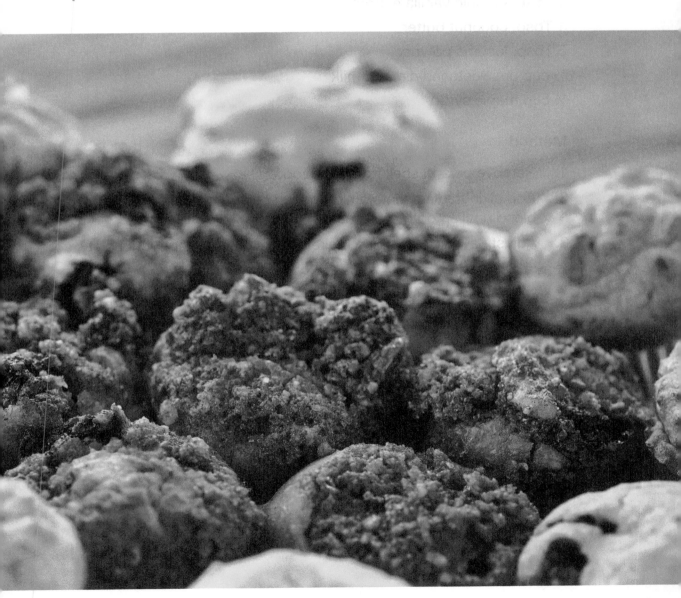

CACAO AVOCADO LUCUMA ICING

Ingredients

3 ripe bananas

2 ripe avocados, removed from shell and pitted

5 Tbsp. raw cacao powder

1 Tbsp. organic vanilla extract

1 Tbsp. coconut butter

5 Tbsp. lucuma powder

½ cup unsweetened almond milk

½ cup maple syrup

Method

1. Remove pit and shell from avocado.

2. Add all ingredients into a high-speed blender or food processer and blend until smooth and creamy.

3. Adjust flavour to taste. To make a slight bit sweeter or chocolaty, add another Tbsp. of lucuma powder or raw cacao.

Prep Time 5 minutes   **Ices** about 12-14 regular-sized cupcakes
Keeps chilled in fridge for 2-3 days

CAROB MACA ICING

Ingredients

2 ripe bananas

1 ripe avocado, out of shell and pit removed

3 tsp. lucuma powder

1 tsp. organic vanilla extract

3 Tbsp. carob powder

1 Tbsp. maca powder

1 cup hazelnut butter

2-3 Tbsp. unsweetened coconut milk

Method

1. Remove pit and shell from avocado.

2. Add all ingredients into a high-speed blender or food processer and blend until smooth and creamy.

3. Adjust flavour to taste, to make a slight bit sweeter or more carob tasting add another Tbsp. of lucuma powder or carob powder.

Prep Time 5 minutes   **Ices** about 12-14 regular-sized cupcakes
Keeps chilled in fridge for 2-3 days

CACAO NIB BANANA CAKE

Ingredients

2 cups all-purpose gluten-free flour blend

2 tsp. baking powder

Pinch sea salt

1 Tbsp. cinnamon

½ cup applesauce

3 eggs

1 Tbsp. pure vanilla extract

7 ripe bananas

2 Tbsp. lucuma powder

1 cup olive oil

½ cup cacao nibs

⅓ cup raw cacao powder

½ tsp. ground chia

½ tsp. ground flax meal mixture

2 tsp. boiling water

Method

1. Pre-heat oven to 375 degrees Fahrenheit.

2. Grease a 9x9 baking dish with coconut oil.

3. In a large bowl combine flour, baking powder, cinnamon, lucuma powder, sea salt, cacao nibs, and cacao powder.

4. In a second bowl, mash bananas then add applesauce, eggs, vanilla, and olive oil. Mix well.

5. In a small bowl, mix chia and flax meal with 2 tsp. boiling water and stir into a paste. Add to wet ingredients.

6. Combine dry and wet ingredients then pour into 9x9 pan and bake for 35-40 minutes. Check for doneness when a toothpick comes out clean in the center.

7. Remove and allow to cool.

8. Ice with Carob Maca icing or Cacao Avocado Lucuma Icing and serve.

Prep Time 15-20 minutes   **Bake Time** 35-40 minutes   **Makes** 12-16 pieces of cake, depending on size

CACAO COCONUT ICING

Ingredients

½ cup coconut butter

3-4 Tbsp. lucuma powder

1 Tbsp. vanilla

½ to ¾ cup unsweetened almond milk

2-3 Tbsp. raw cacao powder

Method

1. Combine all ingredients in a high-power blender or food processor and blend until smooth.

2. Put icing into fridge to cool for 10-15 minutes.

3. Add a bit less liquid for a thicker icing.

4. Depending how much chocolate you like, play around with more or less cacao and lucuma powder.

Prep Time 5 minutes   **Ices** about 10-12 regular-sized cupcakes
Keeps chilled in fridge for 2-3 days

CHERRY CACAO NIB GRANOLA BARS

Ingredients

2 cups gluten-free oats (Only Oats is a good option)

½ cup raw, organic, unpasteurised honey

¾ cup coconut oil

1 tsp. organic vanilla extract

½ cup cacao nibs

¼ cup shredded unsweetened coconut

¼ cup chopped dried cherries

1 Tbsp. cinnamon

Method

1. In a medium-sized pan heat coconut oil and honey. Mix together well, until simmering.

2. Turn off heat and add in all other ingredients then mix together well.

3. Pat out mixture into a 9x9 baking dish until flat and even.

4. Keep in fridge for about 20-30 minutes, then cut and serve.

Prep Time 10 minutes   **Bake Time** 5 minutes   **Makes** 12-14 bars

CHEWY GINGER COOKIES

Ingredients

2 ¼ cups gluten-free all-purpose flour

1 Tbsp. ginger

1 tsp. baking powder

½ tsp. ground chia

½ tsp. ground flax meal mixture

2 tsp. boiling water

1 ½ Tbsp. cinnamon

2 tsp. allspice

Pinch of Himalayan sea salt

1 cup coconut palm sugar

1 egg

1 Tbsp. unsweetened coconut milk

¼ cup blackstrap molasses

¾ cup olive oil

1 tsp. baking soda

1 Tbsp. coconut oil

Method

1. Pre-heat oven to 350 degrees Fahrenheit.

2. Add flour, ginger, baking powder and soda, cinnamon, allspice, sea salt, and sugar into a medium-sized bowl and mix well.

3. Add egg, coconut milk, molasses, and olive oil to a separate medium-sized bowl and mix thoroughly.

4. In a small bowl add chia and flax meal with 2 tsp. boiling water and mix into a paste. Add to wet ingredients.

5. Combine wet and dry ingredients and mix well until a ball of dough is formed. Adjust spices to taste.

6. Chill in the fridge for 15-20 minutes.

7. Grease 2 cookie sheets with coconut oil.

8. Roll cookie dough into walnut-sized balls and use a fork to flatten cookies.

9. 12 cookies fit nicely on each cookie sheet.

10. Bake for about 10 minutes.

11. Cool and serve.

Prep Time 20 minutes   **Bake Time** 10 minutes   **Makes** 24 cookies

CHILI CHOCOLATE PUDDING

Ingredients

4 ripe avocados

7 Tbsp. raw cacao powder

4-5 Tbsp. lucuma powder

1 Tbsp. organic vanilla extract

½ cup unsweetened coconut or almond milk

½ cup dark grade maple syrup

1 tsp. chilli powder

Method

1. Remove pit and shell from avocado.

2. Add all ingredients into a high-speed blender or food processer and blend until smooth and creamy.

3. Adjust flavour to taste—to make a slight bit sweeter add another Tbsp. of lucuma powder.

4. To make it a bit less thick, add more milk.

5. Serve into bowls and top with cacao nibs, coconut or whatever you like.

6. Keeps chilled in fridge for 2-3 days.

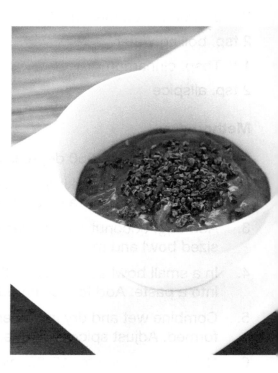

Prep Time 10 minutes   **Serves** 4-5

CHOCOLATE HAZELNUT FUDGE

Ingredients

1 Tbsp. maca

1 cup coconut butter

1 cup coconut oil

4 Tbsp. raw cacao powder

⅓ cup raw, organic, unpasteurised honey

1 Tbsp. organic vanilla extract

½ cup unsweetened shredded coconut

2 Tbsp. lucuma powder

1 cup ground hazelnuts (optional)

Method

1. Tear a large piece of parchment and put into a 9x9 baking dish.

2. Add coconut oil and butter to a medium size pan on medium heat until melted.

3. Add honey, vanilla, lucuma powder and cacao powder and whisk until smooth and creamy.

4. Add coconut and hazelnuts and mix well.

5. Pour over parchment paper in baking dish and freeze for 1-2 hours.

6. Pull off parchment and cut into desired serving sizes.

Prep Time 5 minutes   **Cook Time** 5 minutes

Makes about 12-16 medium-sized pieces of fudge

CHOCO MINT SOFT SERVE

Ingredients

4 bananas out of the peel, frozen

5 Tbsp. cacao powder

1 tsp. pure vanilla extract

2 Tbsp. lucuma powder

2 Tbsp. maple syrup

1 cup unsweetened coconut milk

4 Tbsp. cacao nibs

2 tsp. organic peppermint extract

Method

1. Peel 4 bananas and place in a Ziploc in the freezer until frozen.

2. Add all ingredients except cacao nibs into a food processor or high-speed blender and blend until creamy and smooth.

3. Divide into bowls and top with cacao nibs and mint leaves.

Prep Time 10 minutes   **Serves** 4

LUCUMA VANILLA PIE CRUST

Ingredients

1 ½ cups all-purpose gluten-free flour

1 tsp. organic vanilla extract

1 ½ tsp. lucuma powder

Pinch of Himalayan sea salt

4 Tbsp. cold unsweetened almond milk

½ cup coconut oil

1 tsp. coconut oil

Method

1. Pre-heat oven to 400 degrees Fahrenheit.
2. Combine flour, sea salt, and lucuma powder then mix with a fork.
3. Add coconut oil and blend in well with fork.
4. Add vanilla and milk, then mix crust together.
5. Grease a 10-inch pie plate with 1 tsp. coconut oil.
6. Pat crust evenly into pie plate.
7. Bake for 15-20 minutes, crust only.
8. Add filling and bake for 10 minutes at 400 degrees Fahrenheit, then reduce heat to 350 degrees Fahrenheit for about 35-40 minutes.

Prep Time 10 minutes   **Bake Time** 15-40 minutes, depending on filling or not

Makes 10-12 pieces of pie

OATMEAL VANILLA COCONUT SANDWICHES

Ingredients (For the cookies)

1 ¼ cup coconut palm sugar

¼ cup lucuma powder

1 cup olive oil

1 egg

1 ½ cups gluten-free oats or quinoa flakes

¾ cup shredded unsweetened coconut

2 tsp. pure vanilla extract

1 ½ cups gluten-free all-purpose flour

1 tsp. baking soda

1 tsp. baking powder

1 Tbsp. cinnamon

½ tsp. ground chia

½ tsp. ground flax meal mixture

2 tsp. boiling water

1 tsp. coconut oil

Ingredients (For the vanilla coconut filling)

½ cup coconut butter

3-4 Tbsp. lucuma powder

1 Tbsp. vanilla

½ to ¾ cup unsweetened almond milk

Method

1. Pre-heat oven to 350 degrees Fahrenheit.
2. Mix olive oil, coconut sugar, and eggs.
3. Add oatmeal, coconut, and vanilla. Mix well.
4. Add flour, baking powder and soda.
5. In a small bowl, mix chia and flax meal with 2 tsp. boiling water and stir into a paste. Add rest of the mixture and mix well.
6. Grease 2 cookie sheets with coconut oil.
7. Roll into walnut-sized balls and flatten with a fork.
8. Bake for 15 minutes, then cool on cooling rack.

9. In the meantime, combine coconut butter, lucuma powder, vanilla, and almond milk in a high-speed blender or food processor. Place in the fridge for 10-15 minutes.

10. Once cookies have cooled, spread a tablespoon of icing onto each cookie and top with a second cookie for sandwiches!

Prep Time 20 minutes   **Bake Time** 15 minutes   **Makes** 12 sandwiches

OLD SKOOL COCONUT OATMEAL COOKIES

Ingredients

1 ¼ cup coconut palm sugar

¼ cup lucuma powder

1 cup olive oil

1 egg

1 ½ cups gluten-free oats or quinoa flakes

¾ cup shredded unsweetened coconut

2 tsp. pure vanilla extract

1 ½ cups gluten-free all-purpose flour

1 tsp. baking soda

1 tsp. baking powder

1 Tbsp. cinnamon

½ tsp. ground chia

½ tsp. ground flax meal mixture

2 tsp. boiling water

1 tsp. coconut oil

Method

1. Pre-heat oven to 350 degrees Fahrenheit.
2. Mix olive oil, coconut sugar, and eggs.
3. Add oatmeal, coconut, and vanilla then mix well.
4. Add flour, baking powder and soda.
5. In a small bowl, mix chia and flax meal with 2 tsp. boiling water and stir into a paste. Add rest of the mixture and mix well.
6. Grease 2 cookie sheets with coconut oil.
7. Roll into walnut-sized balls and flatten with a fork.
8. Bake for 15 minutes and allow cookies to cool before moving them off cookie sheets.

Prep Time 20 minutes   **Bake Time** 15 minutes   **Makes** about 24 cookies

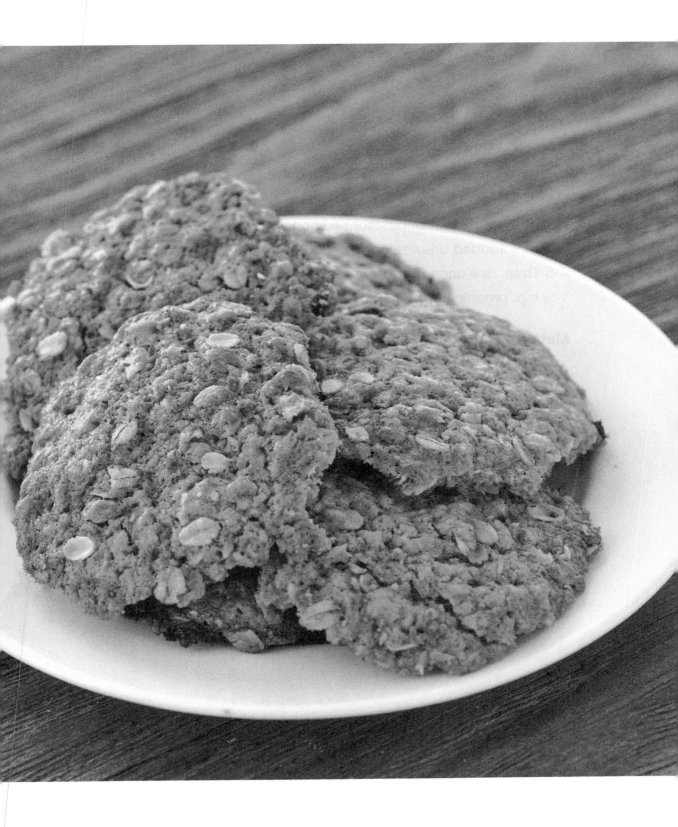

PEPPERMINT CHOCO COCONUT FUDGE

Ingredients

1 cup coconut oil

1 cup coconut butter

1 Tbsp. pure vanilla extract

½ cup lucuma powder

½ cup organic, raw, unpasteurised honey

½ cup shredded unsweetened coconut

4-5 Tbsp. raw cacao powder

1 ½ tsp. organic peppermint extract

Method

1. Tear a large piece of parchment and put into a 9x9 baking dish.
2. Add coconut oil and butter to a medium-sized pan. Place on medium heat until melted.
3. Add honey, vanilla, lucuma powder, peppermint extract, and cacao powder. Whisk until smooth and creamy.
4. Add coconut and hazelnuts then mix well.
5. Pour over parchment paper in baking dish and freeze for 1-2 hours.
6. Pull off parchment and cut into desired serving sizes.

Prep Time 10 minutes   **Cook Time** 5 minutes   **Makes** about 12-16 pieces of fudge

PUMPKIN SPICE COOKIES

Ingredients

1 can organic pumpkin

1 ½ Teff Flour

Pinch of Himalayan Sea Salt

1 cup Maple Syrup

½ cup olive oil

1 tsp. Vanilla Extract

1 cup smooth almond butter

½ cup pumpkin seeds

4 tbsp cinnamon

1 tsp. nutmeg

Method

1. Pre-heat over to 350 degrees Fahrenheit
2. Combine flour, sea salt, cinnamon, nutmeg and pumpkin seeds in a large bowl
3. Combine maple syrup, olive oil, vanilla and almond butter in a high speed blender or food processor and mix until smooth and creamy
4. Mix wet ingredients in with the dry and mix thoroughly
5. Take 2 large pieces of parchment and cover 2 cookie sheets
6. Drop batter by tablespoon onto the parchment
7. About 12 cookies per cookie sheet fits well
8. Bake for 17-20 minutes or until cookies are golden on top (take a peek at the underside of the cookies if they are golden brown they are done.

Prep Time 10-15 minutes   **Cook Time** 17-20 minutes

Makes about 24 cookies

PUMPKIN SPICE FUDGE

Ingredients

1 can organic pumpkin

1 Tbsp. pure vanilla extract

½ cup maple syrup

1 ½ Tbsp. cinnamon

1 tsp. nutmeg

1 cup coconut oil

1 cup coconut butter

2 ½ tsp. pumpkin spice

Method

1. In a medium-sized pot, over medium heat, melt coconut oil and coconut butter.

2. Whisk in vanilla, maple syrup, and pumpkin until smooth and creamy.

3. Add cinnamon, nutmeg, and pumpkin spice, adjusting flavour to taste.

4. Pour over parchment paper in baking dish and freeze for 1-2 hours.

5. Pull off parchment and cut into desired serving sizes.

Prep Time 10 minutes   **Cook Time** 5 minutes
Makes about medium-sized pieces of fudge

PUMPKIN PIE

Ingredients (For the crust)

1 ½ cups all-purpose
gluten-free flour

1 tsp. organic vanilla extract

1 ½ tsp. lucuma powder

Pinch of Himalayan sea salt

4 Tbsp. cold unsweetened
almond milk

½ cup coconut oil

1 tsp. coconut oil

Ingredients (For the pie filling)

1 can organic pumpkin

3 Tbsp. coconut oil

1 Tbsp. pure vanilla extract

3 eggs

Pinch of Himalayan sea salt

4 Tbsp. cinnamon

2 tsp. pumpkin spice

1 tsp. nutmeg

1 Tbsp. gluten-free all-purpose flour

4 Tbsp. organic, raw, unpasteurised
honey

2 Tbsp. coconut palm sugar

Method

1. Pre-heat oven to 400 degrees Fahrenheit.

2. Combine flour, sea salt, and lucuma powder. Mix with a fork.

3. Add coconut oil and blend well with fork.

4. Add vanilla and milk. Mix crust together thoroughly.

5. Grease a 10-inch pie plate with 1 tsp. coconut oil.

6. Pat crust evenly into pie plate.

7. Meanwhile, add all ingredients for pie filling into a high-speed blender
   or food processor and blend until smooth and creamy. Adjust spices
   and sweetness to taste. If you like more of something, add a bit more!

8. Pour filling into pie crust.

9. With filling, bake for 10 minutes at 400 degrees Fahrenheit and then
   reduce heat to 350 degrees Fahrenheit for about 35-40 minutes.

10. Let pie cool for about 15-20 minutes and serve with Vanilla Coconut
    Icing and a sprinkle of cinnamon on top!

Prep Time 20 minutes   **Bake Time** 35-40 minutes   **Makes** 10-12 pieces of pie

PUMPKIN SPICE MUFFINS WITH CINNAMON CRUMBLE

Ingredients (For the muffins)

2 cups all-purpose gluten-free flour

3 eggs

½ cup olive oil

2 tsp. vanilla

2 Tbsp. cinnamon

1 tsp. pumpkin spice

½ cup coconut sugar

2 tsp. baking powder

1 ½ tsp. nutmeg

Pinch sea salt

1 cup apple sauce

1 cup organic pumpkin

½ cup unsweetened coconut milk

½ tsp. ground flax meal mixture

2 tsp. boiling water

1 tsp. coconut oil

Ingredients (For the cinnamon crumble)

½ cup coconut oil

1 cup ground pecans

1 tsp. sea salt

½ cup coconut sugar

1 Tbsp. cinnamon

Method

1. Preheat oven to 375 degrees Fahrenheit.

2. Add flour, baking powder, cinnamon, nutmeg, pumpkin spice, coconut sugar, and sea salt to a medium-sized bowl and mix.

3. Add milk, eggs, olive oil, applesauce, vanilla, and pumpkin into a separate bowl and mix thoroughly.

4. Combine chia, flax, and boiling water in a small bowl, then mix until thick.

5. Combine wet, dry, and chia-flax mixtures together until batter is smooth.

6. Take 2 mini-muffin trays and add paper liners.

7. Spoon batter into muffin trays.

8. Combine all ingredients for cinnamon crumble into a bowl and mix well.

9. Spoon cinnamon mixture over the top of each muffin to cover surface.

10. Bake for about 23-25 minutes.

11. Test with a toothpick and when it comes out clean they are ready.

Prep Time 20 minutes   **Bake Time** 23-25 minutes   **Makes** 38 mini muffins

RASPBERRY CACAO HEMP CUPCAKES

Ingredients

2 cups gluten-free all-purpose flour

1 Tbsp. pure vanilla extract

⅓ cup hemp seeds

½ cup apple sauce

4-5 Tbsp. raw cacao powder

Pinch Himalayan sea salt

1 ½ pints raspberries, rinsed and dried

¾ cup olive oil

1 Tbsp. apple cider vinegar

2 tsp. baking powder

1 Tbsp. lucuma powder

½ cup maple syrup

3 eggs

¼ cup cacao nibs

¼ cup raw unpasteurised honey

Method

1. Pre-heat oven to 375 degrees Fahrenheit.

2. In a large bowl combine flour, hemp seeds, cacao powder, sea salt, baking powder, lucuma powder, and cacao nibs.

3. In a medium-sized bowl combine vanilla, applesauce, olive oil, apple cider vinegar, maple syrup, eggs, and honey. Mix well with a whisk.

4. Combine wet ingredients with dry, mix well, then add raspberries.

5. Line 2 mini-muffin tins with 24 muffins each and fill liners with batter.

6. Bake for 18-20 minutes, and check if done with a toothpick in center.

7. Cool, then ice with an icing of choice. I love the Carob Maca Icing.

Prep Time 20 minutes   **Bake Time** 18-20 minutes   **Makes** 48 mini muffins

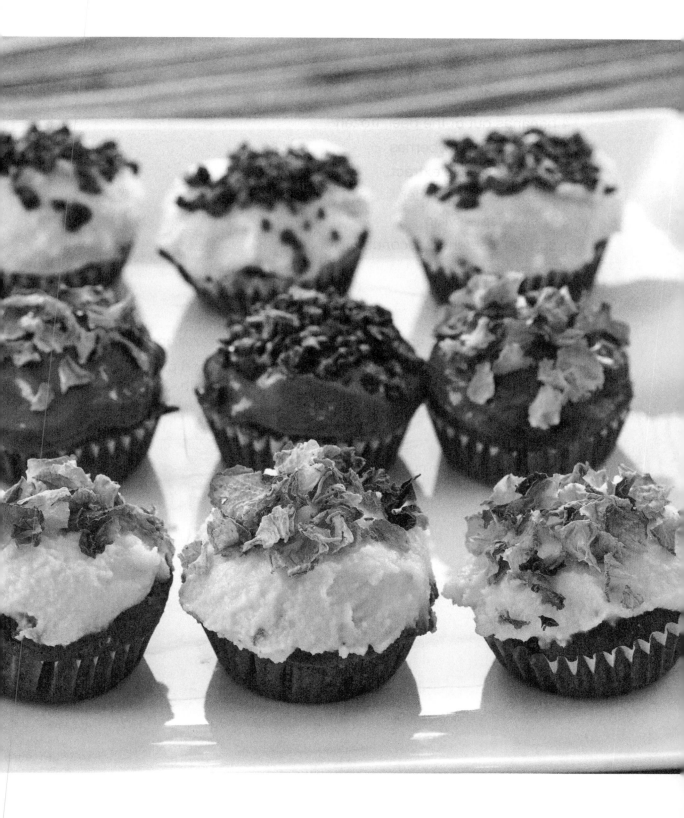

STRAWBERRY BANANA SOFT SERVE

Ingredients

4 bananas out of the peel, frozen

1 cup frozen strawberries

1 tsp. pure vanilla extract

2 Tbsp. lucuma powder

2 Tbsp. maple syrup

1 cup unsweetened coconut milk

4 Tbsp. cacao nibs

Method

1. Peel 4 bananas and place in a Ziploc in the freezer until frozen.
2. Add all ingredients, except cacao nibs, into a food processor or high-speed blender and blend until creamy and smooth.
3. Divide into bowls and top with cacao nibs.

Prep Time 5-10 minutes   **Serves** 4

SWEET POTATO FUDGE

Ingredients

1 can organic sweet potato

1 Tbsp. pure vanilla extract

½ cup raw, unpasteurised honey

¾ cup raisins

½ cup crushed pecans

2 Tbsp. cinnamon

1 cup coconut oil

1 cup coconut butter

Method

1. In a medium-sized pot, over medium heat, melt coconut oil and coconut butter.

2. Whisk in vanilla, honey, and sweet potato until smooth and creamy.

3. Add cinnamon, pecans, and raisins, adjusting flavour to taste.

4. Pour over parchment paper in baking dish and freeze for 1-2 hours.

5. Pull off parchment and cut into desired serving sizes.

Prep Time 10 minutes   **Cook Time** 5 minutes
Makes 12-16 medium-sized pieces of fudge

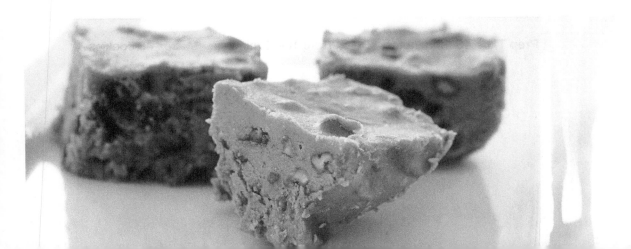

TEFF CHOCOLATE HAZELNUT COOKIES

Ingredients

3 cups teff flour

Pinch sea salt

1 cup dark grade maple syrup

1 cup olive oil

2 tsp. organic vanilla extract

2 cups hazelnut butter

1 cup of cacao nibs or vegan chocolate chips

Method

1. Pre-heat oven to 350 degrees Fahrenheit.
2. Combine flour, sea salt, and chocolate chips in a large bowl.
3. Combine maple syrup, olive oil, vanilla, and hazelnut butter in a high-speed blender or food processor and mix until smooth and creamy.
4. Mix wet ingredients in with the dry and combine thoroughly with hands until dough forms a large ball.
5. Take 2 large pieces of parchment and cover 2 cookie sheets.
6. Roll dough into walnut-sized balls and flatten with a fork.
7. About 12 cookies per cookie sheet fits well.
8. Bake for 10-12 minutes (take a peek at the underside of the cookies if they are really brown they are done.)

Prep Time 10-15 minutes   **Bake Time** 10-12 minutes   **Makes** 48 cookies

VANILLA COCONUT CREAM ICING

Ingredients

½ cup coconut butter

3-4 Tbsp. lucuma powder

1 Tbsp. vanilla

½ to ¾ cup unsweetened almond milk

Method

1. Combine all ingredients in a high-power blender or food processor and mix until smooth.

2. Put icing into fridge to cool for 10-15 minutes.

3. Add a bit less liquid for a thicker icing.

4. Adjust flavour to taste, if you want a bit more of a maple flavour add more lucuma.

Prep Time 5 minutes   **Ices** about 10-12 regular-sized cupcakes

Keeps chilled in fridge for 2-3 days

VANILLA CUPCAKES

Ingredients

2 cups gluten-free all-purpose flour

Pinch sea salt

2 tsp. baking powder

¼ cup and 2 tsp. coconut palm sugar

¼ cup lucuma powder

3 eggs

½ cup unsweetened almond milk

2 tsp. pure vanilla extract

1 cup apple sauce

½ cup olive oil

1 Tbsp. honey

1 tsp. cinnamon

½ tsp. ground chia

½ tsp. ground flax meal mixture

2 tsp. boiling water

Method

1. Pre-heat oven to 375 degrees Fahrenheit.

2. In a large bowl combine flour, coconut palm sugar, sea salt, baking powder, lucuma powder, and cinnamon.

3. In another bowl combine eggs, almond milk, vanilla, apple sauce, olive oil, and honey

4. Combine chia with flax in a small bowl and add boiling water, mixing until thick.

5. Combine wet, dry, and chia-flax mixtures together until batter is smooth.

6. Take 2 mini-muffin trays and add paper liners.

7. Spoon batter into muffin trays.

8. Bake for about 16-17 minutes.

9. Let cool and then ice with Vanilla Coconut Cream Icing and top with cinnamon.

Prep Time 20 minutes   **Bake Time** 16-17 minutes   **Makes** 48 mini muffins

CPSIA information can be obtained at www.ICGtesting.com
Printed in the USA
LVOW02s0708140415

434506LV00001B/1/P